HOLISTIC BODYWORK FOR PERFORMERS

a practical guide

Janet Free and Nicky Ramsay

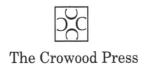

The Crowood Press

First published in 2004 by
The Crowood Press Ltd
Ramsbury, Marlborough
Wiltshire SN8 2HR

www.crowood.com

British Library Cataloguing-in-Publication Data
A catalogue record for this book is available from the British Library.

ISBN 1 86126 699 5

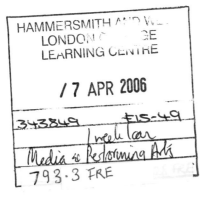
Typeset by Jean Cussons Typesetting, Diss, Norfolk

Printed and bound in Great Britain by CPI Bath

CONTENTS

DEDICATION

This book is dedicated to all our teachers who have made it possible:

Jane Fenwick
Garet Newell
Nik Kyriacou
Wataru Ohashi
Sonia Moriceau
Dick McGraw
Andrew James
Bill Wood
Maxine Tobias
Chungliang Al Huang
Julia and Laurie Lovelle
Peri Aston
Anja Saunders
Suzannah and Ya'Acov Darling Khan
Barbara Ferrier

Our thanks go to Ghislaine Granger at Told by an Idiot, Farooq Chaudhry for Akram Khan, Rebecca Hanson for Russell Maliphant and Jo Phillips at Shakespeare's Globe Theatre who generously supported with photographs.

Grateful thanks to Jan Rosser for creative illustrations and Roy Cook for all model photos. Our gratitude goes to colleagues and students past and present at St Mary's College, Strawberry Hill, who have responded with such creativity to our experimentation, and especially Jo Machon for her insightful comments.

We are also indebted to the following: Laura Pannack, Hilary Pannack, Tina Bicât, Susan Burke, Ulick Burke, Alun Raglan, Deborah Steel, Marco Prado, Alison Jeffers, Mary Clare McKenna, Maxine Doyle, Mojisola Adebayo, Moira Packer, Ruth Derbyshire Moore, Sam Fenton, Mark Fadula, Eloise Carr, Katy Pearson, Gemma John Lewis and Lauren Ramsay.

And finally our beloved, supportive partners, Neil and Davey.

All line drawings by Jan Rosser.

Model photographs by Roy Cook with additional photos by Janet Free and Laura Pannack.

PREFACE

More than a hundred years ago Stanislavski 'discovered' the benefits of yoga for the acting process, yet this is not the aspect of his work that he's best remembered for. In the West we are more likely to celebrate intellectual discoveries. Other cultures, particularly in Asia, have long regarded the body and mind as being in a mutual relationship where neither functions successfully without connecting to the other. In the West we are only just beginning to rediscover the wisdom of the body, as complementary therapies become more mainstream. It is now becoming commonplace in any rehearsal room to find yoga or other bodywork practices going on. Increasingly, it is recognized that our ability to function creatively as performers can be enhanced by developing a holistic connection between body and mind, which acknowledges that the two are inseparable.

It is the aim of this book to share some holistic body practices and to show how they can stimulate the creative process in the theatre. Through these techniques we hope to achieve the 'available' body. This is a body that is open and can articulate clearly without tension. It is grounded yet alert; one that volunteers for action without inhibition or conceit. We begin by looking at 'hard' and 'soft' bodies. By releasing the body armour, which can be both emotional and physical, we discover 'body memory'. This extraordinary resource can then be unlocked in our quest to activate the expressive body. The threefold experience of melting, discovering and transforming contains the essence of holistic bodywork to performance.

The chapters are organized around central concerns of the performing body and suggest a range of specific bodywork practices with practical suggestions for experimentation. There is an introductory chapter on getting into the reluctant body followed by chapters on recovering the child-like body; discovering the yin and yang within us; sourcing energy channels; learning to take risks through disorientation; grounding; and finally using breath to bring the body and mind into a state of readiness for performance.

The bodywork practices begin with the Alexander Technique that originated from attempts to remedy the effects of performance-related stress. It is now a highly popular body alignment approach for musicians and actors in theatres and academies across the world. Feldenkrais is a lesser known approach to bodywork that encourages a powerful release of the entire being through simple, repeated exploratory movements. Tai chi and yoga have certainly become important, not just in rehearsal rooms, but also in spas and retreats worldwide. Shiatsu and reflexology offer opportunities to explore the body's energies and healing powers through touch. Contact Improvisation is a movement form that encourages immediacy of performance response by releasing and trusting the body, thus developing spontaneity and intuition. A principal focus in achieving the connection between the body and the mind is through the breath. This is dealt with in the final chapter uniting all the practices. Breathing is giving life to performance: it is the dynamo and inspiration for expression. All of the practices introduced here are valuable in their own right but have special applications to performance.

Some of the very real benefits for performers of working through the holistic body are as follows:

- discovering the power and potential of breath to connect body and mind;
- recognizing your own habits and learning how to let go of surface tension;

- building up your energy/stamina/strength reserves to be able to survive the pressures of rehearsal and performance;
- developing a sense of grounding and centering;
- appreciating how emotion memory is locked in the body and finding out how it can be sourced and used creatively;
- discovering the value of touch to nurture interaction;
- opening up to new experiences that make you creatively braver;
- learning to trust and follow your instincts;
- encouraging bonding and ensemble commitment;
- developing your own physical vocabulary so that you can be more articulate on stage.

These practices may be of special interest to devotees of physical theatre but will also be beneficial to performers, directors and teachers working through other forms of theatre, music and dance. Whatever the style of performance the body is always paramount. Whatever the style of body the holistic connection is always paramount. The older and larger body can be just as magical in action as the lithe and athletic. These practices are for all bodies - whatever the shape, size, flexibility, age or capacity. Exercises are set out with careful instructions to avoid injury, but caution should be taken to work in clutter-free environments, with matting if possible, and with safety in mind.

The book will start you off working in a more holistic way with exercises for individual practice, and partner work to engage in touch and discovery that will prepare you for creative experiences. As each bodywork practice is encountered you will find a brief overview giving information on its origin and key characteristics. If you want to deepen any particular bodywork practice you can follow this up by using the contact information at the back of the book. Our exercises are merely an introduction and should in no way be regarded as a substitute for professional classes and individual tuition. However, performers are by nature magpies. This book gives you an opportunity to try out some of the possibilities for holistic practice, a worthwhile investment at any level. One of the values of the book lies in its comparative approaches and the way in which it draws evaluative connections between the different disciplines. Besides stimulating creativity and raising awareness and expressivity of the body, these experiences can bring real benefits for protecting the performer's wellbeing.

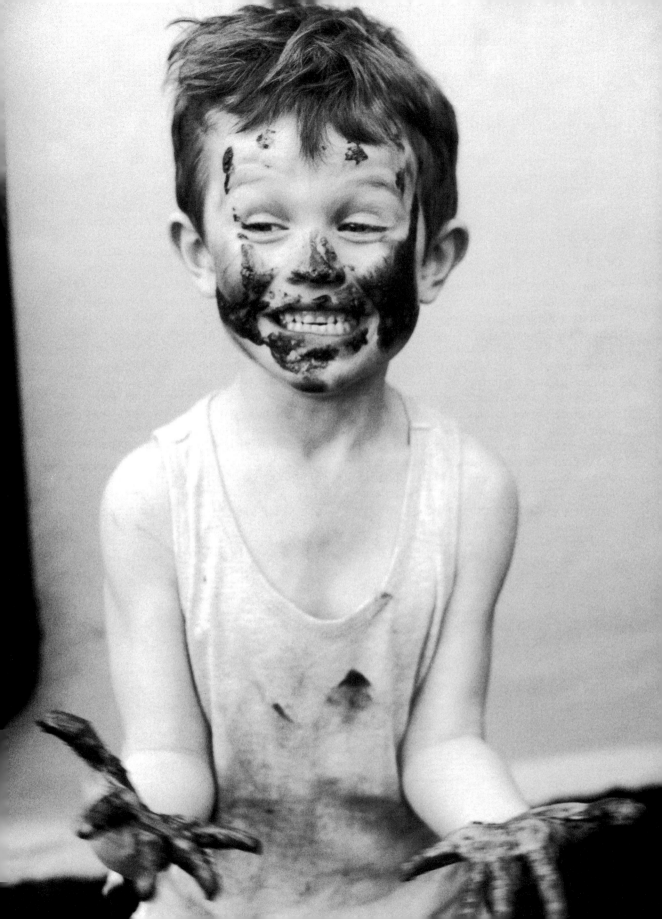

1 MELTING THE BODY'S SEAL

THE PARADOX OF PERFORMANCE

Performance is a heightened state of live contact that energizes and transforms. The adrenaline rush that accompanies such an intense act of communication takes us to places beyond the everyday. Yet so often when the body primes itself for performance we find ourselves tightening up as we become conscious of being in the spotlight. The more we try to control our bodies with the head, the more sensations of stage fright are liable to find their way to the surface and let us down. Para-doxically, this moment of performance, when our bodies need to be most ready, is the very time when they are often most reluctant. The performer's body needs to be strong to deal with the pressures of performance, yet at the same time it also needs to be vulnerable and yielding to be able to express itself with sensitivity. The toughness of the profes-sion means that you have to become thick-skinned to survive and yet what is required for creativity is openness. The challenges begin at the rehearsal stage when we need to get in contact with our bodies and to break through the protective seal with which we have held ourselves together for years. In order to do this we have to work to erase layers of tension before we can really listen to our bodies and hear the stories they have to tell.

ADULT BODY/CHILD BODY

In the adult body the senses become dulled and less spontaneous yet what is remarkable when watch-ing a child at play is how all the senses seem to be alive. There is a wonderful quality of exuberance

and lack of inhibition. As we get older we learn to behave. This leads to a restriction on our bodies as we contain ourselves both emotionally and physically. Before we know where we are, we are editing ourselves, holding back and acting out. This has a profound effect on our body language. Studies have shown that children use up to 50 per cent more space around themselves in self-expression than their adult counterparts.

As we grow, we subconsciously pick up patterns of behaviour by adopting standardized body language and so pressures of conformism can tend to affect the freedom of our body movement. We think of how uniforms standardize the body and

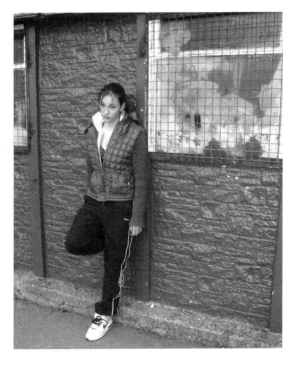

Adolescent 'attitude'.

*OPPOSITE: **No worries.***

prevent the individual retaining their sense of identity. This is evident in the military where rigidly upright postures can seem very forced. However, this kind of conditioning also occurs in very different cultural contexts as young people succumb to the influences of media and peer groups. Look at the way the teenage girl on page 11 stands expressing her adolescent 'attitude'.

It is often in our adolescence as we develop sexual self-consciousness that we try to protect ourselves by concealing the self. With the onset of puberty, people become uncomfortable with their bodies and ill at ease with their growing selves. Even those who have apparently emerged from the adolescent slump and slouch may retain feelings of discomfort in relation to certain areas of the body. A sense of inadequacy and disconnection from self can often be made even worse by media images dictating how we should look. This can make us even more self-conscious. Alternatively there is the opposite response – that is, to be overconfident with our bodies and strike flamboyant 'actorly' poses. This is just as much a self-protective attitude as one of shrinking withdrawal. These attitudes are an inevitable part of social survival that the sensitive performer needs to learn to unravel in order to arrive at a neutral place from which to begin their own physical expressivity. Along the way, in rediscovering their own authentic body expression, it can be valuable for the performer to recognize the subtle forms of body language that reveal levels of public masquerading. These observations can provide a source of fine characterization in theatre work. First of all though, they must be aware enough to appreciate what is going on in their own bodies, beyond the obviously physical.

BODY ARMOUR

Infancy provides a marvellously carefree and protected environment for our bodies. It is a time when we are not afraid of falling and don't think too much about the consequences of our actions. As we grow, we encounter checks on our sense of adventure and curiosity; we learn to withdraw ourselves and develop caution. Every time we face

a threatening situation we build up more and more layers of tension that eventually develop into visible 'holding' patterns, forming what we might call a *body armour*. Rounded shoulders, tightly held jaws, rigid walking styles and so on, are all manifestations of what can be called *psycho-physical* responses to the world, as emotional experiences leave their physical imprint on the body. Sometimes the outward expression of tension may not be obvious but can be subtle and almost hidden, such as the scrunching up of toes or even internal tensions such as headaches or irritable bowel. Our bodies' defence mechanism against trauma is to cut us off from the feeling in order to protect us. As a result our bodies can be left numb and insensate. The creative process requires that we have a free passage between our senses, our movements and our body memories.

MELTING THE BODY

There are many different ways of helping ourselves to get us into our bodies when we are feeling particularly disconnected or stuck. We could choose to take an exuberant, playful approach, helping us to release energy and reconnect with our inventive selves. Directors and practitioners have long known the value of games and play, some ideas for which are given below. Alternatively, we can help to break the body's seal by melting tension with a reflective mind/body approach and later in this chapter we will be exploring some sensitized bodywork exercises. First though, some playful, 'recovering the child activities', which can be very useful in reminding us of our spontaneous and gleeful selves. In practice, what works well in any rehearsal regime is a combination of each of these kinds of activities, adapting the mix according to the specific needs and experience of the group and the material you are working on. Sometimes, if the energy is low or the work demands it, you may want to start with some game playing. At other times, after a long, intensive bodywork session and to bring the company back to a sense of the present, a game may be the thing to help us return to the here and now after some demanding internalized work.

RECOVERING THE CHILD EXERCISES

Thinking back to your childhood self, what differences do you notice about the way you inhabited your body then and how you do so now? What differences do you notice in energy, pace, use of space, spontaneity/control? Do you have any specific memories around physical play, such as sliding down banisters/stairs, wrestling/mock battles with siblings, rolling down hills, water/mud/snow play? Share experiences of these with a partner and try to say which of these spurts of childlike physicality made you feel most alive. Have a go at skipping with a rope, doing a handstand, or a headstand on the sofa, cartwheeling down hills, playing with puddles, kicking leaves. If we find these exercises undignified, or feel slightly silly, this is probably very revealing and tells us something about how we have lost contact with our childhood sense of play. If you can, remind yourself of what it's like to play a childhood game. Remember 'stuck in the mud', 'wink murder'? Ideally, play these outside as you probably did when you first enjoyed them and try to recapture that in-the-moment quality.

What is sometimes productive, if you are doing character-based work is to play the games in role. This is doubly beneficial since you get all the benefits of the game-playing for yourself plus the chance to make interesting discoveries about how your character behaves and interacts with others.

FROM THE PHYSICAL TO THE KINAESTHETIC

Probably you are already familiar with strategies like warm-up games as a means of getting more physically dynamic and open. This book attempts to take us beyond that purely external level towards a sensory awareness that will help develop a sixth sense, beyond the conventional five, known as the kinaesthetic. This does not refer to the supernatural but is about a heightened sense of the body in space that extends to our feeling of what is going on within. The naming of this sense that has been described as the 'eyes of the body',

Pre-Rehearsal Games Are Good For:

- Energizing the body and keeping fit and lively.
- Recovering a lost sense of exuberance.
- Reviving imagination and inventiveness.
- Having fun.
- Making us aware of and enjoying the contribution of others.
- Developing our 'wicked' side – too often lost to the sober correctness of adulthood (If you ever get a chance to play capoeira, a Brazilian martial art/dance form, this idea of a robust sense of 'trickery' is developed to a wonderful degree).
- Refreshing us and giving our 'head-bound' selves a break.

has enormous implications for our ability to both know and express ourselves. The following exercises take us some way towards awakening this kinaesthetic awareness.

Kinaesthetic Body Awareness Exercises

Lying Down

When we first ask ourselves to become aware of the body, it may be that we can't feel anything much at all and this is where it is often helpful to begin by lying on our backs (this is called the supine position). It's the position from which we started off in the world as babies so an excellent place from which to begin a journey of rediscovering our expressive possibilities. In this position, our bodies are undefended and we do not feel the need to try to do or prove anything. Instead of simply noticing our external activity, as we would do if we were on our feet and ready to go, we stand a better chance in supine position of beginning to tune in to what is actually occurring within the body and to use this information to develop an awareness of our inner bodies.

1. The first thing is to find a warm, comfortable place to lie down. Don't lie directly on a cold floor but use a mat and/or layers of blankets to

support and cushion the body. It's really important that we feel the possibility of giving the weight to the ground. Lie down carefully and have a sensation of letting gravity look after your body weight. Begin to pay attention to the curves of the body and the places where it makes contact with the floor and where there are spaces. There are three natural curves at the neck, waist and knee. Don't try to force these to flatten, but you may notice as you release more into the ground that a degree of sinking has taken place.

2. As you begin to let go and to soften the outer body, take the attention into the breath and get to know the inner body landscape. Think about the passage of the breathing, the weight of the bones and the oxygen pulsing to every cell. Notice in particular how the weight of the head, and the shoulder and pelvic girdles gradually becomes heavy and naturally wants to sink towards the ground.

Six Limbs
From this supine position, take the arms over the head and slowly begin to stretch your limbs one at a time, exploring the space around you, keeping contact with the ground. Conventionally, we think of our limbs as being confined to our arms and legs but now close your eyes and try to imagine that your head and your tailbone are additional limbs with their own motion. Just as the spine is the first part of the baby to grow, imagine that your body is back in the cocoon of the womb, making its first explorations of the space around it. Play with a sense of rolling and writhing as with each breath, the limbs reach further. Explore the space in the air above the body. It is helpful to have some ambient music playing, maybe based on the sounds of nature.

Breathing Through the Feet
Remaining on your back, bring the knees up and have the feet flat on the floor so you are now in semi-supine. Imagine you are breathing in through the soles of the feet. Follow the passage of the breath into the body, through the lower limbs and into the trunk, before you exhale the breath

through the crown of the head. Repeat five times trying to increase the length of the breath with each round. As you breathe in, keep the belly soft and allow the breath to inflate the chest and rib area so you get a sense of width and breadth on the back of the body. As you exhale, allow the abdomen to deflate, as the belly button draws nearer the spine and the body lengthens and releases on the outward breath. As you repeat this breathing exercise you will gain a sense of contact with the internal body and begin to feel the relationship of the legs through the trunk and to the head.

Body Scan Drawing
Have next to your mat/blanket a large sheet of paper, crayons and pencils for use later.

A valuable starting point for increasing self-awareness is to do a *body scan* drawing exercise. Having completed the breathing through feet work in semi-supine, now allow the legs to stretch out onto the floor and have their full length. From this position, imagine the body is lying in sand and forming an imprint. Be conscious of the weight of the body as it surrenders to the soft warm texture of the sand. Now, from the feet moving upwards towards the head, try and have a sense of the right and left sides of the body. Is one leg rolling out and giving more weight to the ground than the other, or is one buttock more in contact? Do the shoulders feel equal or is one flatter to the ground, the other more raised? What is happening with the head? Don't be tempted to adjust the position or make judgements on your body alignment but just for now observe what is going on and keep breathing through each area of the body as your attention moves into that part.

Start to register what you feel about your body and how that affects your own body image. The tensions that are held are imprints of your experiences so that in tracing your body you are also getting in touch with how you respond to it. How do you wear your body to the rest of the world? Inevitably, this exercise may throw up discomfiture or anxieties about the body but it is likely to give us valuable insights into our *body signature*, alerting us to areas of the body where we need to accept, embrace and learn to release a little more! Next time you lie down you will do so with an improved kinaesthetic knowledge.

Having scanned the body in this way, now slowly bend your knees and roll over onto one side, before coming up. Take up your pens and paper and without thinking about it too much begin to draw what you feel about your own body. You don't have to picture the whole body but if you are feeling particularly aware of, for example, your shoulders or your ankles, your drawing may register a magnified image of these areas. Be aware of any injuries or significant experiences that may have affected the sense of your body's outline. What you should aim for is to let your picture show graphically, and in any way you choose, the areas of your body that are particularly strong in your own consciousness.

After this initial reflection, it is useful to begin to bring sensation in to the body and each of the following yoga-based exercises helps us to feel the connection between different body parts.

Kinaesthetic Awareness Exercises
Yoga-Based Knee to Chest Sequence

1. Begin by lying on the back with knees drawn up in what is called the semi-supine position. Take an inhalation. As you exhale draw one knee into the chest and lightly hold the shin.

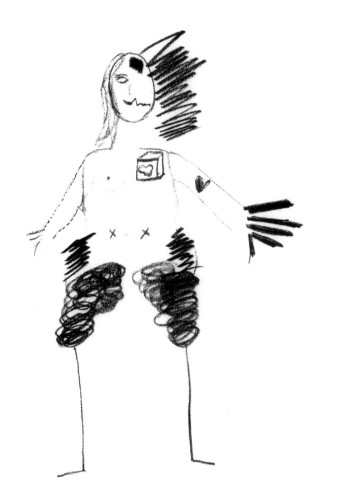
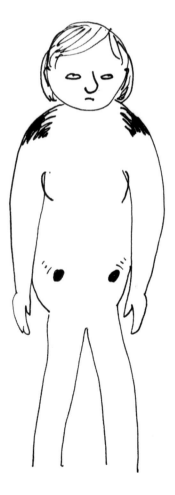

Body scans revealing subjective responses.

2. Inhale raising same leg to ceiling. You can hold the leg with the hands to help it to stay upright. Try and keep leg straight even if you can't keep it perpendicular.

3. Release the grip and lower the leg exhaling it down to within an inch of the ground. As you do so, stretch the heel away from the ground. Keep leg held in this position as you inhale again before beginning the cycle once more, exhaling the bent leg towards the chest. Repeat five times.

4. Before you move to other leg to repeat the exercise, return to semi-supine and rest in this position. Notice the difference in the way your lower back feels on the side you have just been working. There should be a far greater sense of ease, and the connection of pelvis and trunk will feel much more released.

This exercise brings kinaesthetic awareness to hips and spine using the breath.

Yoga Sequence – The Moving Bridge

1. Begin in semi-supine. Start with a few breaths repeating the breathing through the feet exercise described on page 14. Exhale.

2. Inhale as you slowly lift the lower spine up off the floor and continue to roll the back up through the spine until the weight is supported on your feet, shoulders and head. As before,

really allow the ribs to expand sideways as you breathe in. Time the inhalation to coincide with the movement. You should arrive at shoulder level at the same time that you reach maximum inhalation.

3. Breathe out, reversing the action by lowering the spine, vertebra by vertebra to the ground. As you exhale, sense that the navel and lower abdomen is sucking down and in towards the spine and this will lengthen the waist. Try to time the breathing so your spine arrives at ground level as you finish the exhalation.

4. It may take a few rounds of the sequence to be able to time the breathing to synchronize with the movements. When you have found the right rhythm there is a wonderful sense of rolling up each vertebra of the spine on the breath. It's a little like playing the keys of a piano, making sure that each note is sounded and heard. Repeat five times.

5. When you have learned to time the movements with the breath add the next level of the exercise, which is to work the arms into the sequence as follows:

   Start with arms on the floor beside the body. As you go into *the moving bridge*, raise the arms into the air and allow them to arrive at floor level behind your head as you reach maximum inhalation. As you exhale, float the arms back down to the ground, by your sides.

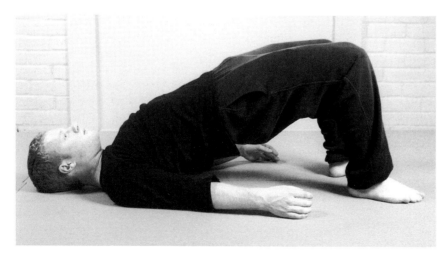

Yoga sequence – the moving bridge.

This sequence brings kinaesthetic awareness to the whole spine through the breath

Yoga Sequence Rotations

The following exercises are carried out in a seated cross-legged position. Sit on a slight thickness (a block or a large thick book) so that the back can remain long and lifted. Lightly hold the feet with the hands.

Stage 1

1. Inhale keeping a sense of the length in the neck and spine.
2. Exhale dropping the chin to the chest.
3. Inhale returning the head to centre.
4. Exhale dropping head back and opening the mouth slightly to release the jaw.
5. Inhale as you return the head to centre.

Repeat five times, then try the following variation:

Stage 2

1. Exhale, tilting the head to the right, allowing the ear to come close to the shoulder but keeping the shoulders soft.
2. Inhale returning the head to centre.
3. Exhale tilting the head to the left, allowing the ear to come close to the shoulder but keeping the shoulders soft.
4. Inhale.

Repeat five times.

Stage 3

1. Centre yourself again in the sitting position and take a couple of breaths. Lift spine, and inhale keeping the shoulders relaxed. Rotate your trunk over your right thigh. As you begin the exhalation, have a sense of a gold crayon on the crown of the head and draw a large circle in the air with the crown of your head, dropping the trunk and head down towards the right side and then sweeping the torso down in front of the body, and through to the centre.

2. When you reach the centre point begin to inhale again, returning the body up through the left side, remembering to rotate the trunk to the left to ease the movement on the way back as you return to the sitting position. Be careful to synchronize the breath with the movement (*see* the illustration overleaf).

Repeat three times starting on the right and again three times starting on the left. It may feel easier to release the hold of the hands on the feet and lightly connect the hands to the floor shifting from side to side as you rotate the upper body around the lower body. Don't worry if at first the circle of your 'crayon' in the air is quite small. These will get larger as the hips and the spine soften and release with the breath of the movement bringing renewed kinaesthetic awareness.

Hard and Soft Bodies

We often aspire to be superfit and feel that a heavy exercise programme is an appropriate way of preparing ourselves for performance. Contemporary approaches to training the body, like aerobics or weight training, may develop the body mechanically but are not always helpful in securing the mental release that's required by the performer. These methods can increase tension and make the body short and tight, rather than lengthened and released. Even forceful yoga regimes, can be counterproductive. Stamina is tremendously important but there are dangers in treating the body like a machine if we submit it to an unmindful pounding. People in this state are often as inexpressive and full of tension as those who don't engage in physical activity at all. These are hard bodies whose armour is so tight that there is no space for being in touch with the internal self. The hard body is a goal-oriented body in which targets achieved in the gym or in competition become more important than the process involved in getting there. When we really listen to the body there is a mutual communication between body and mind, whereas the hard body is controlled largely by the mind. One of the keys to this

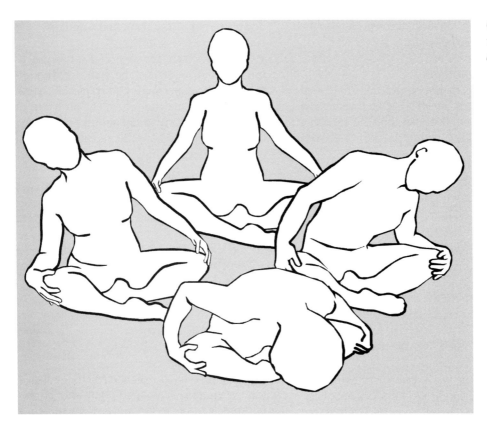

Crayoning with the crown.

dialogue between internal and external is an awareness of the breath.

A simple way of telling whether or not the approach to your body is hard or soft is to try the following stretch exercise. A lot will depend on the nature of the language you use to direct the movement, which has an effect on the way the body perceives the communication and therefore on the quality of the action.

Hard Stretch
1. Stand tall, feet hip-width apart. Raise the arms to the side and stretch them away from the trunk as strongly as you can.
2. Push the arms apart and try to push the fingertips as far away from the centre as possible.

Soft Stretch
1. Stand tall, feet hip-width apart. Breathe in. Exhale, taking the arms away from the body.

Continue to breathe deeply and with each exhalation release the arms away from the centre a little more. Have a sense of the limbs melting away from one another by allowing the shoulders, elbows and wrists to soften and lengthen.
2. Think of the muscle falling away from the bone and take the attention into the fourth finger rather than the middle one. Allow the thought that the arms are extending out of the centre rather than flexing rigidly.

Perform both these stretches and notice which feels most familiar. You may notice that the hard stretch involves frustration, force and tension, whereas the soft stretch involves a sensitised form of releasing the body and finding length, using the breath and being aware of resisting unnecessary muscular effort. If the hard body seeks end-gaining, getting to a fixed destination as quickly as possible, then the soft body is about feeling one's

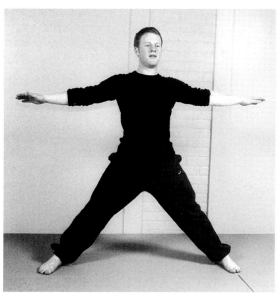

Hard stretch.

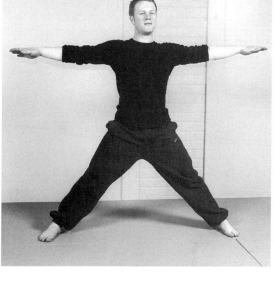

Soft stretch.

way into the pose. The *thinking body* is one that feels transparent and alive rather than stuck and solid. When we talk about the soft body that's not to say that it should be floppy and lifeless. There needs to be a potential dynamism even within a relaxed body; the image might be of a slumbering cat that can spring to life at a moment's notice. This ideal of the body that is soft, open and responsive is very desirable to any meaningful creative performance work.

As demonstrated in the hard and soft stretch exercise above, the key to discovering the soft body is through the breath. Try the following partner breathing exercise that may help to unlock a bound body.

Breathing Exercises: Partner Hands on Back

This exercise may be done with your partner sitting or standing but is best achieved lying on your stomach on the floor. This is called prone position.

1. Take a few moments to become aware of your partner's breathing. Gently place the palm of your hand on your partner's back wherever you feel an instinct to do so. It is important not to think about it but to feel the area to which your hand is attracted.
2. Let your hand rest there for a minute or two and encourage your partner to breathe into your hand. You may feel heat or tension in that area or it may be that the area feels lacking in energy. Your own 'breathing hand' can help draw your partner's breath to soothe tension or energize weak areas. Continue using both hands resting on the back to encourage deep breathing. Take as much time as you need before swapping over.

This exercise may take a while to tune into. It is important to go with your instincts and not get agitated if you don't get immediate results.

Body Memory

Body memory is a phrase describing how our experiences imprint themselves on and in our bodies. The memory exists not in our conscious mind but in the form of sensations held deep in the tissues of the body. For at least a century now,

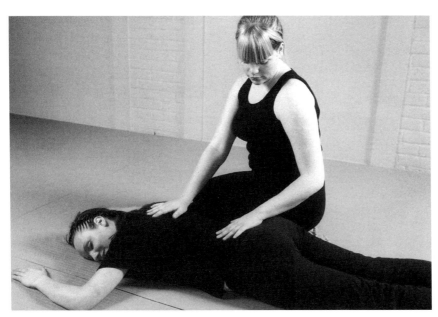

The breathing hand.

performers and theatre makers have recognized that the body is a repository of emotional history. This is particularly evident in visibly bound bodies in which self-expression is difficult because emotions are locked in. Freud and other psychoanalysts recognized the crucial connection between mind and body and at an early stage realized that the way to reach the subconscious mind was through relaxing the body (on the couch!) Their work on the idea of powerful experiences being rooted deep in the body memory, formed the basis for Stanislavski's own ideas on emotion memory. He very quickly saw its potential for personal creativity. He realized that the key to authentic performance was the actor's willingness to engage with these sensations and to use them to re-experience important emotional states in the creation of character. Any of the exercises in this chapter would provide a strong basis on which to prepare the body for Stanislavski's emotion memory work.

Because we live in a world that places a great premium on being rational and in control, we often learn to suppress our emotional and sensory selves. We may not even be conscious that this repository of feelings and sensations exists until we begin to breathe underneath the surface of our inhibitions. Holistic bodywork can provide a way of retrieving the valuable creative resource of body memory by helping us to be more in contact with the (sensate) place where our bodies and emo-tional memories intersect. Unfortunately, many directors approach the excavation of emotional memory from a purely mental angle whereas the whole point is to create a *holistic* pathway that brings together body, mind and emotion. This approach is much more likely to bring about a physical communication in performance. Various bodywork innovators have experimented with methods to help the body soften, open and recover a natural expressiveness and in the early twentieth century one of the most significant contributors to *psychophysical* awareness was the Australian performer Alexander. At the same time that Alexander was experimenting on his own body/mind use in Australia, the actor and director Stanislavski had been making discoveries about the *psychophysical* in Russia. Both these men were responsible for transforming the nature of actor training.

THE ALEXANDER TECHNIQUE

F. M. Alexander (1869–1955) was an Australian classical actor who repeatedly lost his voice during performance. After observing and analyzing his own body use, he realized that under the stress of performance he was in the habit of stiffening his neck, which resulted in a restriction in his throat causing his voice to become strained. His habitual misuse of the body was exaggerated in the performance situation. Realizing that the head–neck relationship was the crucial area in releasing tension throughout the whole body, he developed a method of relearning how to use his body. He did this by simply rediscovering how to do very ordinary activities such as walking, sitting, standing and lying with a free neck. He realized that by only using the minimum amount of muscular effort, the body would perform in a more effective way that avoided holding tension. Having cured his own vocal problems he worked through hands-on teaching, helping actors and singers to improve their vocal and body use. His method became known as the *Alexander Technique*. As his teaching expanded, discoveries of the benefits went beyond the acting profession as the improved breathing and body use brought positive effects to people's general health. It soon spread further afield to the medical profession and the sporting world. Today, people all over the world benefit from his technique and it is now commonplace to find Alexander teachers giving classes in body use at all the leading Drama Schools and Music Academies as well as the larger theatres and opera houses. Just as sporting teams have a support staff of physiotherapists, large theatre companies have Alexander teachers to help actors prevent injury and maintain good use of the body, particularly vital when the body has to deal with the relentless demands of performance.

To really understand the method it is vital to receive hands-on private tuition to sense your own habits and experience the guidance of the teacher redirecting your body use. This is a worthwhile investment, not just for performance, but for the rest of your life. You can still gain some benefits from group sessions and from your attempts to

The Main Principles of Alexander's Teaching

- *Recognition of habit* – becoming aware of how we misuse our bodies.
- *Primary control* – the observation of animals' use of lengthened spine and head-led movements and applying this principle to our own *use.*
- *Inhibition* – a moment of pause that enables one to prevent the habit before it has the chance to reoccur. (Note that this is not the Freudian more conventional use of the word 'inhibition' that indicates a closing up of feelings).
- *End-gaining* – becoming engaged in the process of movement and action rather than being preoccupied with achieving a goal.

Alexander's Cardinal Directions are that: *The neck should be free so that the head can go forward and up and the back lengthen and widen.*

These Directions do not just refer to the physical direction of movement but should grow out of visualization of the action. It is often enough simply to visualize the *direction* in the mind in order to bring about a change in the body rather than crudely imposing a different state on the body. This is very revealing in terms of what it tells us about the power of the mind–body connection.

increase awareness through reading but all these exercises will be a lot more meaningful after even just a few sessions with a professional.

End-Gaining

Alexander noticed that many people lead their lives thinking constantly about the future and not being grounded and living in the present. Terms like 'head in the clouds', 'up in the air' and 'thinking ahead' are suggestive of how our heads may be disconnected from our bodies and not conscious of what is going on around us. Our tendency to force things to be done is often shown in activities such as driving, playing computer games and chopping

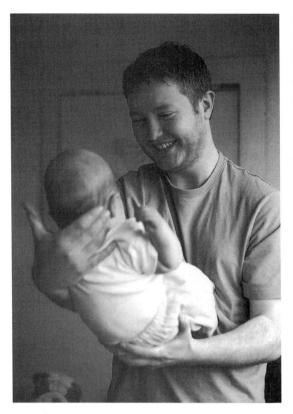

Good body use.

contraction. By doing this for the recommended 20 minutes a day you will allow your spine to regularly lengthen and help the rest of your body build up a sensory awareness by which it will feel tensions in the body and act to erase these. You may have to start with 5 or 10 minutes but try eventually to build up to 20 minutes. It takes this long for gravity to have a significant effect in allowing the vertebrae to release, and the discs in between the vertebrae to recover from the contraction imposed when upright. The body in this position will lengthen by several centimetres as the discs that are like little sponges, regain their elasticity. Think of it as plumping up the cushions that have become flattened.

vegetables. We tend to tense up and concentrate on the product and not the process, an attitude that he termed 'end-gaining'. Through a heightened awareness of what is going on in the body, second by second, Alexander's technique really focused on the need to be present in the moment and not to 'end-gain'. You could think of it as stopping to smell the roses. This results in less tension and wasted energy and a much more sensory appreciation of life going on around us, which is hugely beneficial for performers. The idea of being *in the moment* is very much associated with Zen philosophies and there is a strong connection between the 'less is more' notion of Eastern philosophies and Alexander's work.

Semi-Supine

This is the basic Alexander position from which to learn to rest your spine and try to prevent

1. Start by finding a book on which to rest your head. It needs to be about 4 or 5cm thick. Place it at one end of a yoga mat or blanket on the floor. Now you need to get down to the floor by keeping your neck free and spine long so kneel first and then get into a seated position on the floor. Now lower your spine down slowly so that your head comes to rest on the book. This provides an important function in supporting the back of the skull so that the curve of the top part of the spine, the neck (cervical vertebrae), can spread out. Make sure the book only touches the back of the skull so that the neck is free to lengthen.
2. Make sure that your knees are raised and your feet are planted firmly on the ground. Your knees should ideally be in line with your hips. Let your back settle naturally so that your lower back is in greater contact with the floor. You may still feel a gap between the floor and your lower back but this will subside over time with practice. Think of allowing your spine to lengthen, and widen your shoulder blades like spreading your wings.
3. Be careful not to allow your jaw to tilt up and cause the neck to bend. Think of your jaw sinking towards your chest. Place your hands over your stomach above your hips and think of your fingers spreading and softening.
4. In this position try to bring your attention to the different parts of the body and check that

Semi-supine.

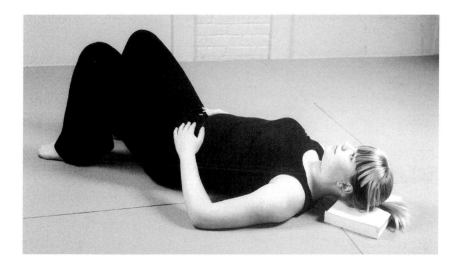

you are allowing all those tight muscles to uncurl. It is helpful to think in terms of the spiralling action of the muscles winding around the bones, so visualize an unravelling taking place and a softening of the joints. Try visualizing honey or warm olive oil seeping through the ankles, knees and hips and shoulders.

It is important to do the semi-supine position on the floor and not on a bed or a couch as you need to be on a hard surface for gravity to work on the spine. Your body also responds to the magnetic fields of the earth. It is a very nurturing position to be connecting with the earth, although at the beginning you might feel quite vulnerable when doing this.

At the end of the exercise, with the head released, roll over onto your side with the head leading and the body following the spiral movement. Resist the impulse to bring the legs first and let them follow on. Get up onto your knees, rolling up the spine from the pelvis to the neck. Now step up onto your feet keeping your neck free, head forward and up and back wide and long.

Wandering Minds

For some people the moment they lie in supine, a million and one thoughts go dashing through their minds and they are unable to focus on the exercise in question because they can't get their heads to connect with their bodies for a sustained length of time. This is quite common as we live in a culture in which there is a continuous flow of information and we are constantly on the go. We are not practised in meditation where the mind and body are brought together. In fact, for many people 'down time' often means collapsing their body on a sofa while the mind is entertained by TV. If your mind wanders and jumps as you do your Alexander lying down, then you can try the following:

1. Listening – close your eyes and listen to the sounds around you. You may be aware of the loudest and most immediate but try to extend beyond this to the more subtle background sounds and noises in the far-off distance. Make sure that the breathing is soft as you gently continue to listen. After you have done this for 3–5 minutes you can then open your eyes whilst still listening out for every noise. Hopefully this will have opened up that sensory perception and helped you to remain in the moment.

2. Visualization – focus on your breathing by using a visualization. Imagine that there is a little hole in the middle of your chest and as you inhale you are drawing in a golden light that fills up your chest. Hold onto the breath for

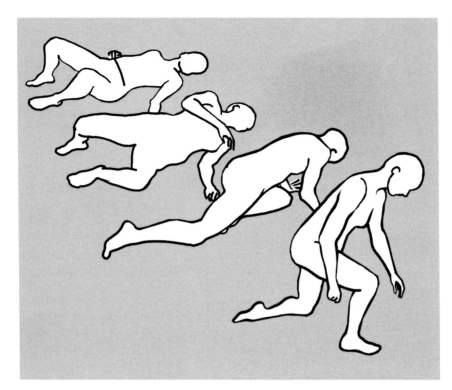

Head leads from floor to standing.

a few seconds and feel the golden warmth inside you. As you exhale, follow the breath as it travels up through the throat and fills the entire head and then wafts away through a little hole in the crown of the head. You can repeat this, imagining that the hole is in the navel and fills the stomach and then exhaling the breath through the feet.

3. Body Monitoring – bring your attention to each part of your body in turn to monitor where there is tension. You can start at the feet and work up the body but take your time to really feel what is going on in each area and to think of softening. Bring your awareness not only to your muscles but also to the bones and joints. You should breathe into each area.

If you are experiencing lower back pain then it is counterproductive to keep lying down in a state of tension. Reduce your time and try to build up again to the twenty minutes. If, however, you are only feeling a slight discomfort in your lower back as it

gets used to releasing, bring your knees up to your chest and hold onto them. Then rotate the knees slowly both clockwise and anticlockwise to massage that lumbar area. This will give you a breather. Weaknesses in the lower back will often indicate that the stomach muscles are also weak. The exercise Yoga Knee to Chest Sequence shown at the beginning of the chapter provides a very good way of strengthening these muscles so you could do some of these exercises daily to help tone this area.

If your legs feel like collapsing then perhaps you are not planting your feet firmly enough on the ground and you may need to adjust your alignment, even if it means not quite having your legs parallel with your hips. Bring your heels up closer towards your buttocks. Remember that you need to be breathing into the feet and feeling the contact with the ground.

Standing and Sitting
One of the keys to understanding how our bodies

may move more effectively is to identify where the hinge mechanisms are. The head neck hinge of Alexander's primary control is seen to be the most important. In addition hinges occur at the hips, shoulders, knees and elbows. However, our spine is not a hinge mechanism even though we often treat it as such by slouching and bending. The only spinal joints that are flexible are in the neck (cervical) and lower back (lumbar) rather than the middle spine (thoracic) that is joined to the ribcage, so the vertebrae here tend to get constricted with overuse at either end of the spine. As we do the simplest of movements it is crucial to notice the process or as Alexander termed it 'the means whereby' we perform actions and not try to end-gain.

Aligning the Spine in Sitting

1. When sitting, you should try to maintain a lengthened spine by making use of your sitting bones (ischia) in your bottom. Imagine that they are like little feet that can support you. When you start to enjoy the awareness of these little feet you can expand your back much more easily.
2. Take your bottom right to the back of the chair and put your hands under your bottom to feel your sitting bones. Now get a partner to help you feel your hinges in your hips. Ask them to place their fingertips on the front of your hipbones. Using this resistance, incline your torso forwards hinging from the hips and keeping the back long. Don't forget your *directions* (neck, head, back). Think of a sliding action as the thighbone moves backward to allow the pelvis to move forward. This grounds you in your sitting bones and helps your lower back to feel stronger.

Sitting to Standing

1. Sit with your feet firmly on the ground and your legs at 90 degrees to the floor. If you are short then you will need to move to the edge of the chair to achieve this connection with the floor.
2. You need to sink your weight into your feet, free your neck, bend from the hips so that the

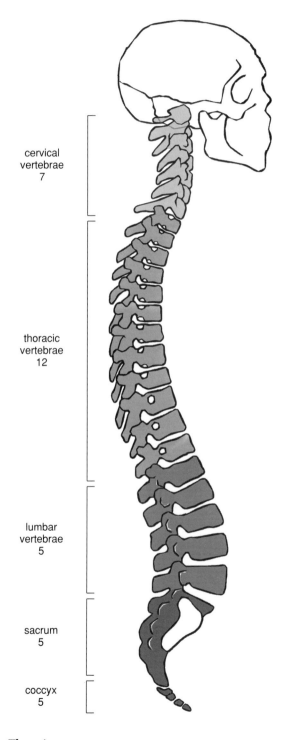

cervical
vertebrae
7

thoracic
vertebrae
12

lumbar
vertebrae
5

sacrum
5

coccyx
5

The spine.

25

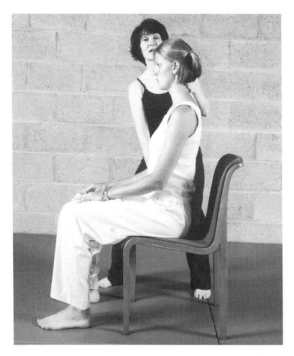

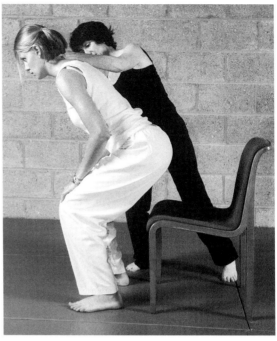

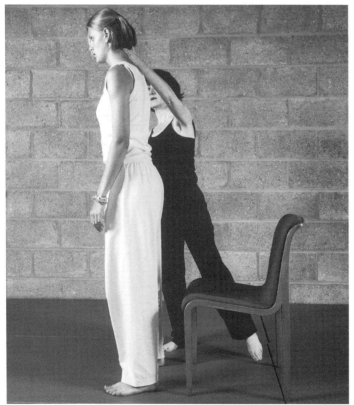

Sitting to standing with Alexander Directions.

weight transfers to the feet and you are able to tilt the body forward effortlessly onto the feet whilst keeping the neck free and the spine long. The forward momentum of the body leaning forward from the hip carries the weight from the sitting bones to the heels. You need to keep the arms loose at the side so that they do not engage in pressing down on the thighs or chair. The work needs to be done by the large muscles in the leg and not involve tension in the back or neck.

Once you start to practise this technique you may feel some discomfort, especially if you sit without slouching for a period of time. This pain is what Alexander calls 'unreliable sensory feedback'. It feels painful so it feels wrong. However this is not the case. It is just that your body has become so accustomed to your habit of slouching or even a rigid upright position, that it feels unfamiliar. You may have lost sensitivity in your postural muscles that you are now activating in the process of realignment. Just for once the dictum 'no pain, no gain' may be right.

Improving Sitting

Work in pairs with one observing and the other doing. The observer places a light touch with two fingers at the top of the neck where it connects with the back of the skull. This is approximately behind the eyes. Get your partner to tighten their jaw and feel the tension that is created in the back of the neck. Now encourage them to sit and stand with an Alexander awareness. You can quickly identify for them whether or not they are allowing their heads to retract and their jaws to come forward, not just by observing but also by feeling what is happening at the top of the neck. Now try doing the reverse by sitting from standing. Keep the neck free as the knees bend and the body inclines forward from the hips keeping the spine long until the bottom finds the seat of the chair. This can feel quite a distance but your partner will support you until your confidence builds.

Sitting in Performance

When on stage you may have to sit without looking to see where the chair is. Whenever we are cautious about an action the body will tense up and it may be difficult to sit with a sense of our Alexander Directions. However, the body memory functions instinctively if it is given some reminder. If you touch the seat with the back of your leg so that your body knows that it is safe to descend without trepidation, this will release the tension in the head/neck as you descend.

Neck Jazz

This exercise helps release the neck area and provides an enjoyable sensation of freedom in the neck if you are able to surrender control.

1. Work in pairs with your partner lying on a mat or blanket in supine with eyes closed. Kneel at their head, your knees parallel with their shoulders. It is useful to put on some relaxing music and to make sure that your partner is warm.
2. Take their head in your hands but do not lift it off the floor by more than a few centimetres. Just get a sense of how heavy it is. A head generally weighs between 10 and 12lb (4.5kg and 5.5kg), so if you are only getting 6lb (2.5kg) then you need to hold it still for a little longer to try to encourage a sense of trust, so that your partner will release more of the weight.
3. Start to rotate the head from one side to the other, exchanging the head from one hand to the other in a very slow figure of eight. Don't forget to breathe yourself! Many people feel so cautious about touching the head they tend to be a little reverential and tense.
4. Check that your own spine is long, neck free, head forward and up. If necessary, you may need to adjust your position to get a little closer to their body. You are encouraging the chin to move toward each shoulder but do so as gently as you possibly can so that you build up the extension further each time.
5. Should you feel a tightening up do not go any further. If you follow the breath you can encourage more release on the exhalation. Notice if your partner starts to force the movement of the head; many people find it difficult to give up

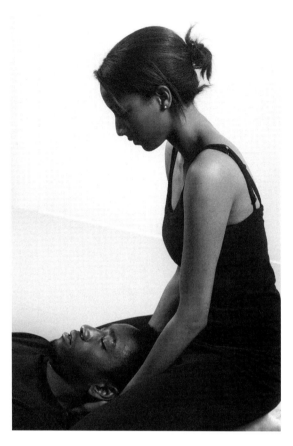

Neck jazz.

control. Just slow down the action even further or change direction. However, there may come a point where the movement becomes a shared action rather than involving a leader and a follower.

6. Once you have built up a flowing movement you may want to extend this into a more improvisatory neck jazz. Keep the movements quite slow but more playful. Try rocking the head slowly back and lifting the head upwards but always mindful of how your partner is responding. What seems a very slow exercise may feel incredibly vivid and dynamic for the person lying down and if you go too fast you are liable to make them feel dizzy. Some slow jazz playing is helpful to set an undulating rhythm.

7. You may feel quite vulnerable after this exercise. As with many exercises that involve releasing control of the body, it may also bring with it a release of emotions that have been held. Always give time for recovery and if necessary a chance for some feedback. For some, this exercise can induce a feeling of flying, whilst for others it can create an uneasiness about relinquishing control.

More Head and Neck Visualization

In Alexander work the Primary Control, head–neck relationship is really the central principle on which the technique is based. As a preparation for the next chapter that focuses on further Alexander work, there are a few helpful ways of encouraging this head/neck release.

1. Stand with feet hip-width apart.
   Visualise the head just balanced on the spine like an apple bobbing on water. Try and have a sense of the head releasing and experiment with tiny movements letting the top of the head lead the movements. Particularly, allow the head to release forward and up away from the neck.
2. An image that might be helpful is to think of a horse with a bridle and reins that is 'given its head'. Like the horse having 'free rein', we should enjoy the sensation of leading with the head free and the jaw soft. We are often 'reined in' by habits and tensions that interfere with our freedom of movement and make us fixed rather than flowing, with jaws locked by reins.

Avoiding Stage Fright

To return to the beginning of the chapter where the deadly effects of stage fright were discussed, a useful technique to employ the second before you are about to perform is to take a step onto the back foot and just pause before going on stage. This is a moment of what Alexander would call 'inhibition' that will prevent you from rushing 'headlong' (the term really encapsulates that jaw thrusting forward).

Recap

Why the Alexander Technique is beneficial for performers:

- Improves body use with better posture, alignment and increased grace.
- Improves breathing and results in wellbeing.
- Increases sensory perception (kinaesthetic awareness).
- Teaches an approach that fosters *being* not *doing.*
- Avoids bad postural habits and performance clichés.
- Encourages a sense of being *in the moment* increasing ability to be spontaneous and creative.
- Encourages a sense of being responsible for our own bodies.
- Builds confidence and combats stage fright.
- Increases awareness of the crucial head–neck relationship that governs body use.
- Develops an awareness of body use that extends beyond the physical to an attitude to life.
- Helps rid the body of fixed postures and develop poise.
- Improves vocal capacity through better head/neck alignment.

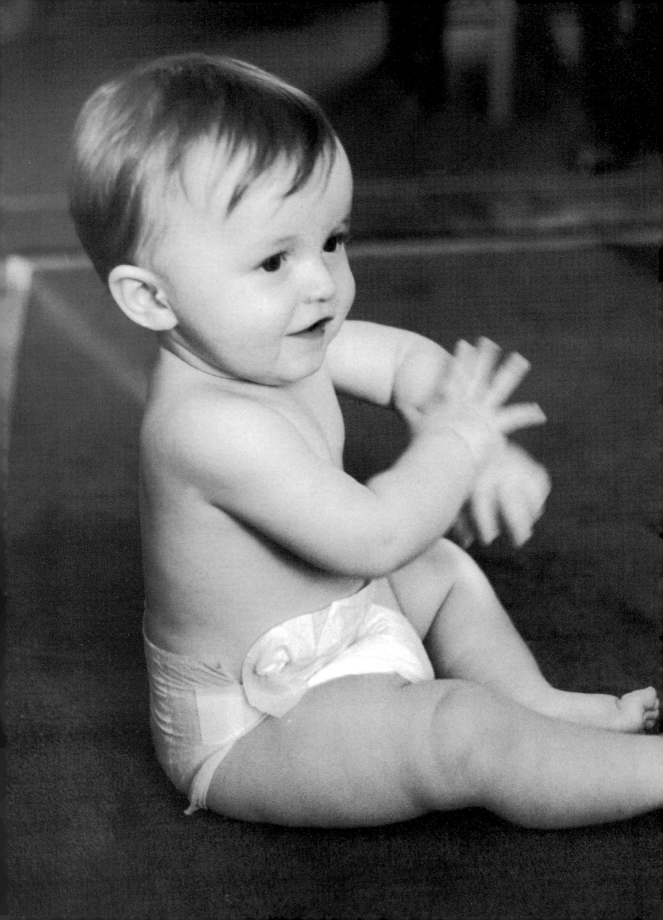

2 THE INNOCENT BODY: MORE ALEXANDER WORK AND INTRODUCING FELDENKRAIS

BEING IN THE BODY

Central to Alexander's thinking about body use is the idea that as adults we may have lost contact with the natural connection we had with our bodies in childhood. The purpose of the 'directions' he developed for the performer and of the Alexander teacher's guiding hands in a typical lesson, is to help remind the body of how it used to feel when in a state of balance and alignment. This concept is to do with *being in the body*, about returning to a state of lightness and grace. This chapter looks at Alexander's work in more detail and explores how to get back to this place of innocent responsiveness. Alongside the exploration of Alexander's work, we introduce the ideas of Moshe Feldenkrais, another visionary who had a lot to say about rediscovering the relationship between the way we feel, think, move and live in our emotions. Like Alexander, Feldenkrais knew that we had much to gain by reconnecting with a child-like sense of discovery both of ourselves and of the world around us. Each of these pioneers had a realization that by releasing the body tensions that prevent spontaneous responses, we could achieve a more open, trusting and intuitive approach to life. In their different ways, both are champions of *The Innocent Body*.

The Neutral Body

The *neutral body* is an expression that comes up a lot in discussions about actor training. In order to

OPPOSITE: *The innocent body.*

arrive at the neutral state of being, it is essential to recover a sense of the innocent body. This helps the performer to let go of the tensions and holding patterns, both mental and physical that interfere with clear and free expression. The neutral state is being balanced, grounded and poised ready for action, with a sensory awareness of what is going on, both inside and outside the body. The neutral body is a desirable place to begin creative work since many of the blocks that interfere with creativity have been dissolved through a return to innocence. The new-found freedom of the innocent body permits an openness of the mind conducive to creativity. The *neutral body* is a state particularly favoured by physical theatre performers who often have to respond to unexpected stimuli, needing to transform into many different likenesses and appearances, unhampered by idiosyncratic mannerisms and personal tensions. Companies and performers in quest of the neutral state have turned extensively to Alexander work and to the Feldenkrais method. Amongst French-trained companies, these approaches are often used in conjunction with neutral mask training as a prelude to various kinds of physical theatre. Feldenkrais work has been absorbed as a vital element in the basic training method for progressive dance companies who demonstrate the extraordinary fluidity and economy of movement made possible by this practice.

Armed Neutrality

One aspect of the neutral body is that it encourages in the performer a state of being *charged* rather

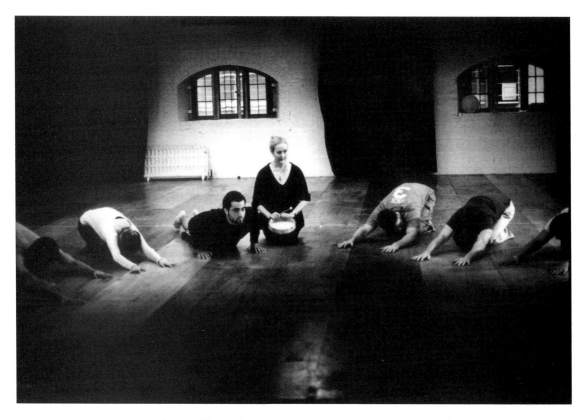

Alexander teacher Glynn McDonald working with student performers at the Globe Theatre, London.
Photograph by Sheila Burnett

than passively inactive. This is a similar state to that sometimes described by martial arts practitioners as *armed neutrality* in which the performer is paradoxically both relaxed yet ready for action at the slightest stimulus. Performers in the process of warming up will often focus on their internal state at the expense of their awareness of the world around them. This can have calamitous results as they become drowsy or glazed, states preventing alert responses. Armed neutrality is about being totally prepared to receive the unexpected and yet retain a sense of the centre. One of Alexander's guiding principles was to develop in the performer an alert curiosity, as if the world and those in it might be approached with a spirit of interest and openness rather than fearfulness.

More Alexander Work
Walking Observation of Others

1. Walk around the circle in a group getting a sense of the way you walk but not concealing any natural tendencies.
2. Pair up and take it in turns to observe the other by walking behind them. Notice any particular postural traits. Does the person bounce as they walk, or hit back with their heels or maintain a creeping action? Do they tilt forward? What kind of pace do they use? Does one part of the body appear to be leading? Is the head held centrally or on one side? Is their head stuck on their neck or freely held? What's going on with the arms and the hips? Are these freely moving or bound, or is one held more than the other? It is important not to be judgemental, but just to

notice what is happening with a sense of interested curiosity.

3. Let them come to rest while you reproduce their walk as accurately as you can. If necessary, slightly heighten any tendencies so that your partner can observe these in action. You will notice a great variety of different walks and holding patterns. This exercise provides much amusement as well as being tremendously informative in making us become aware of our own idiosyncrasies.

4. Swap over and talk about what you have noticed. Now two pairs join up and observe each other's walks and imitations reporting back on how accurately the partners have observed and reproduced each other.

Pink Parachutes – Less is More

Having noted our walking habits, pink parachutes is an exercise that helps us to let go of some of our impulses to push forward and tighten up.

1. Imagine you are trying to walk somewhere in a hurry and think about what your manner of walking might be. What happens to your walking pattern? Do you notice if you are fiercely *end-gaining*, that is concentrating all your attention on the action of arriving rather than journeying. You may tend to lose connection with your body and find yourself pushing your neck forward or tilting your jaw up and compressing the back of your neck.

2. Try it now. Walk around the space with a sense of urgency and notice what this does to your walking pattern. Now try again, and this time put into action a series of thoughts. Instead of putting your intention into where you are going and trying to get there as fast as possible, this time think consciously about being present in the *back* of the body. As you do so, notice how this slows you down.

3. Now, have a visualization that attached to your shoulder blades are a pair of pink parachutes that just gently engage in the wind as they billow out behind you. These instantly affect the way you move forward. You may find

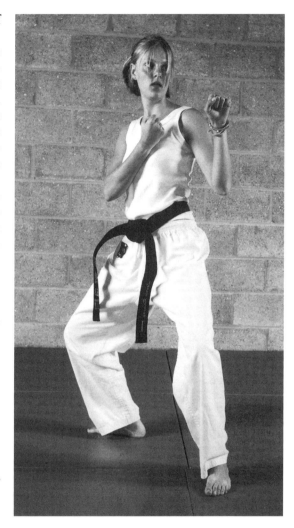

Armed neutrality in martial arts.

yourself slowing down, breathing more deeply, even smiling.

4. Walk again with pink parachutes attached. Always free the neck first. Now feel aware of the space behind and to the sides of you as well as simply focusing on a narrow path straight ahead. We feel more three-dimensional, grounded and spacious. We are likely to feel more present and more connected to our bodies rather than being a disembodied head, making its own crazy way forward.

The Back and Beyond

Pink parachutes should help you begin to sense through the back. This is a neglected area of our sensory awareness as we spend so much time focusing on what is in front of our eyes. You may think of this as you breathe, because the lungs are connected to the back ribs and do not just exist in our front chest. Your awareness of this posterior lung activity will help you breathe into the back. Another useful exercise to do when walking is to think of yourself treading on an imaginary wheel but instead of your legs propelling yourself forward on the wheel, the wheel is actually turning backwards. This visualization, used by Buddhist monks in their walking meditation, is helpful in

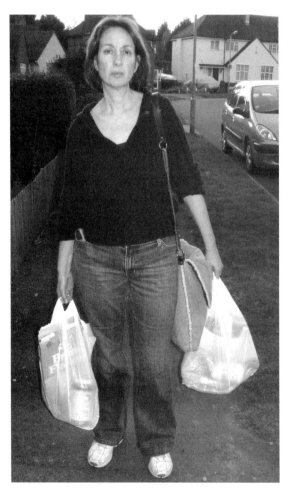

Body bound by unnecessary muscle tension.

discovering a state of poise and equilibrium. The body will immediately respond to the release from forward thrusting by lengthening and elevating. You may also gain more weight in the heels and feel grounded.

Alexander Driving – How Tight Are You Gripping the Wheel?

The Pink Wool Phenomenon

This is another way of thinking ourselves into the back of the body and preventing a headlong rush.

Tie a small length of pink wool onto the steering wheel. Next time you find yourself at the wheel, gripping tightly and shortening the arms, neck and upper body, let the pink wool remind you of the pink parachutes. Breathe, relax and allow more space by softening your shoulders and allowing a sense of length in the arms. You should think of your elbows as being heavy, a thought that might help the arms to release. Run through the Alexander Directions. Remember, free neck, long spine, wide back. Remember also to relax the jaw that can often clamp up at the wheel. Most of the time we're using up vital resources of energy by doing far too much and not being specific enough in our muscle use. If we only call on the precise muscles required to perform any given activity, we conserve energy and prevent fatigue. Alexander has a memorable expression about the strain and overexertion brought on by doing too much – he calls it 'interfering with oneself'. We need to 'leave ourselves alone' (another choice Alexander phrase) and learn to let go of the peripheral muscles. These seem to want to muscle in on any activity, especially those such as driving or per-forming, around which we may have developed anxieties. Often, these secondary bands of muscle never really learn to let go and thus are in a per-manent state of semi-flexion. It is this unnecessary holding that causes us to ache and feel sore, typically in the shoulders, neck, hips and lower back.

Long Arms

It's easy to fall into the habit of using unnecessary tension and shortening our limbs when per-forming everyday tasks, on or off the stage. Next time you are holding a bag, check that you are doing so with a sense of *long arms*, and feel how much easier this is. When your body gets the idea of this approach you will discover that you can do things in this way without exhausting yourself. Make sure you use this principle of length and release when you are on stage. If the character-ization demands tight limbs, then at least do so with a sense of a soft neck – this will protect your own body from the worst effects of bad use. Be sure to make time to unravel after the performance.

Debauched Kinaesthesia

One of the keywords in Alexander work is 'soft-ening'. The technique is about lengthening and widening but not in such a way that the body stiffens or becomes rigid. Another very important concept is that of 'allowing' certain processes and changes to take place in the body, to do with lengthening, releasing and making space within. The simple act of learning how to release the neck by allowing 'the head to move forward and up' permits a miraculous realignment of the body. It also allows for the free flow of certain mental processes. The only way that we can allow ourselves to grow is by recognizing and erasing our bad *habits*, thus giving ourselves the chance to respond afresh to the world within and around us. City living makes us close off physically and emotionally because of known dangers and the need to look out for ourselves. Bad postural habits and stress form part of our response to the risky and competitive world around us. Yet Alexander knew that sometimes habits could be comforting and give us messages of feeling good when the truth may be that these very habits (slouching, shallow breathing, twisted torsos to name a few), merely make us feel safe because they are familiar to us. Sometimes it can feel threatening to open up and soften when we would much rather curl up and protect ourselves with *holding patterns* that we are thoroughly used to. Alexander called this dependence on 'comfy' collapse the state of *debauched kinaesthesia*!

Wooden Performers

When we come to perform and work with

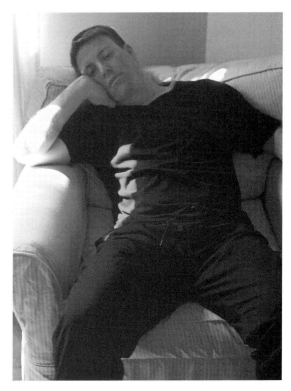

Slouching debauchery!

character, we should ideally be working with a sense of *openness* to allow original work to emerge. Too often however, it is easier to reach for the stereotype because it is ready made and known. A hard body is role-bound – one that reaches for the protection of a stereotype or tricks. Fixed precon-ceptions of character accompany stiffness in the body and the two together make for wooden or predictable acting that is neither inspired nor graceful. Wooden acting holds no surprises and is constructed of cliché. Alexander work encourages the kind of openness that helps us to dodge stereotypes by allowing a lot more space around our creative choices. Instead of reaching auto-matically for a ready-made and obvious perception of character, or other form of expression, an Alexander approach will help us to *inhibit* this response and to take the time and space to allow a more inspiring creative choice to emerge from within.

On the physical side we should also be aware that a fierce adherence to a lengthened neck at all costs can make some Alexander trained actors appear too erect in their posture for roles that require a more contracted body. This fixed ideal body pose is something that is wrongly associated with Alexander as it certainly is not in the spirit of his teaching. This upright pose can seem just as inappropriate as the wooden actor. If the characterization demands tight limbs, then it is really important to convey that on stage but the secret is to do so with a sense of a soft neck to protect the body.

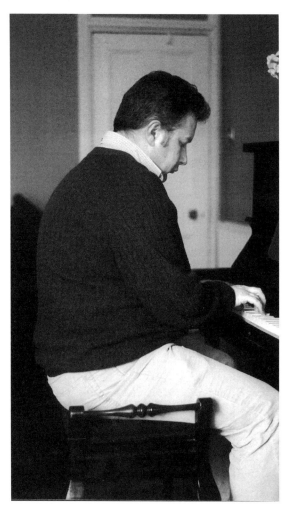

Musician demonstrating poor body use.

Good Use

Musicians, in an effort to hold their instrument in alien body positions, are often in danger of distorting their own body alignment. The same is true about actors and dancers who have to adopt difficult positions for sustained periods during performance. And whilst performers often take the time to warm up for their performance and try to achieve a neutral state in which they can perform in an optimum way, they rarely remember to return their body to the neutral state after their contorted performance. The residues of awkward and unnatural positions stay in the body and develop into areas of pain and misalignment that can become detrimental to future performances. Even in the state of contortion, the damage can be minimized by retaining a sense of the vital head/neck relationship that in Alexander terms is described as the *primary control*. If you are performing in a way that requires you to contort the body, be sure to make time to unravel your body after the performance by doing semi-supine, stretching and getting regular sessions.

More Alexander Space Making

As we have seen, Alexander work is about unfixing the body and making space within. This sense of space is both physical and mental, literally bringing about a feeling of ease and roominess in the body but also allowing the self to spread out into broader creative opportunities. The work begins in the body to make room for the psychological expansion. Below, are a few enjoyable Alexander-based exercises that can help to create this feeling of spaciousness in the body and mind. Since they are all done with a partner, they are also instrumental in nurturing a trusting and sensitive relationship with other company members. Such trust, developing out of an intuitive connection between partners, can be immensely valuable in fostering a strong and healthy ensemble feeling.

Scapular Rest

1. Both partners rest in semi-supine for about five minutes as preparation for this exercise. As you are lying there, remember your Alexander

'directions' and also have a sense of increased length in the arms and legs. Imagine your knees and fingertips extending into space beyond the physical boundaries. The femur (big thigh bone) will feel as if it is infinitely long, extending into space beyond the knee. Both the upper and lower arm bones will likewise feel as though they are projecting out beyond the elbow and fingertips. As the limbs lengthen, there will be an increased sense of space throughout the body. Breathe deeply, observing the changes in the body.

2. Kneel by the side of your partner who remains in the semi-supine position. Push the upper arm of your partner up and away as you insert your left palm under your partner's right shoulder.

3. When the hand is in position beneath their shoulder blade, allow their arm to rest back in the former position.

4. Cup your right hand over the top of their shoulder. Wait for at least three minutes for the shoulder to settle. Both partners breathe deeply and let gravity allow the shoulder joint to continue to fall.

5. When the time is up, keeping the right hand in position on *top* of the shoulder, withdraw your left hand from beneath. This should be quite a struggle if they have really let the joint become heavy. On no account should they help you remove your hand by lifting their shoulder out of the way.

6. Look at the set of their shoulders. The shoulder that has been worked on (the right one) is likely to look far broader, the chest more open. Even the set of the arms will be different with much more room on this side of the body. Repeat the exercise on the other side.

Emperor Concerto – an Alexander-Inspired Movement Duet

This is a popular exercise with those who are developing a kinaesthetic awareness of their body in space and the connection with a partner. It is named after Beethoven's *Emperor's Concerto* (2nd movement), as this seems to work particularly well as an accompanying score.

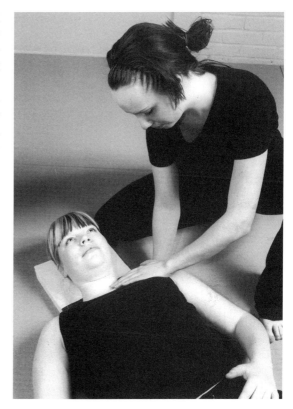

Scapular rest.

1. Stand next to your partner, supporting their left hand in yours and their left elbow in your right hand. Both partners breathe and when you are tuned into your partner's rhythm, the supporter encourages their partner to close their eyes and surrender the weight of their arm. Both partners have soft knees and neck and stand with feet apart to give more stability,

2. Again breathe, and as the music starts, the supporter very gently begins to move the partner's arm, experimenting sensitively with the movements of the various joints. Perhaps start with the fingers and wrist with some gentle rotations and then, if your partner's body seems to be softly unfolding, you can begin to gently extend and play with the movement of their elbow joint. Remember to soften the neck, feeling the connection of the feet on the floor. Keep breathing.

3. As the music continues, take your partner for a short walk and maybe play with the movement of the whole length of the arm. Try taking the arm up high and see if they will allow the shoulder joint to release. Be mindful of all the joints of the arm and ensure that you are always supporting in some way with your own hands.

4. Some pairs develop this exercise into an exquisite movement duet as both bodies shift and extend in response to the changing arm positions. Eventually all the joints will begin to free up. The trick is for the person whose arm is being moved not to anticipate their partner but to wait in the moment for the gentle stimulus that they then follow. Neither resist nor anticipate your partner's movements but allow a subtle dialogue to take place. Do not speak or unduly use eyes, but focus on your kinaesthetic awareness.

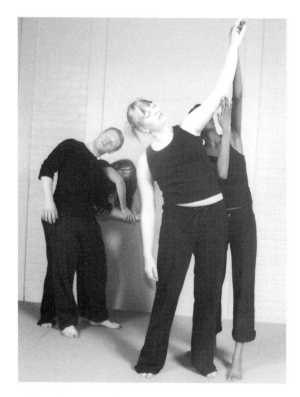

Alexander principles in action in the Emperor duet.

The Alexander Cat

This is a well-known yoga-based exercise, but done here with a head-led, Alexander emphasis it feels quite different, improving what Alexander called our *primary control*. Begin on all fours, on a well-padded mat or blanket to cushion the knees.

1. Breathe in and as you exhale, round the back as you do so, softly curling the neck and dropping the crown of the head towards the chest.

2. Reverse the action but leading with the head as you breathe out, scoop the upper back into a more concave shape. Repeat these movements six times.

3. Both the exhale and the inhale actions should involve the upper rather than the lower part of the spine, otherwise the work is just done on the lumbar spine and the stiffer upper back remains inert. Thinking about the action coming from the head is a much more effective and natural way of performing Cat position (*see* opposite).

Extending the Cat Sideways

The Cat position is a useful one for exploring the developmental patterns of human movement. As babies grow, their movement patterns progress alongside their neurological development. In the womb they are already beginning to flex and extend their limbs yet once they are born they begin to learn how to co-ordinate their actions to move in patterns. The first movement of the spine is the head and tail movement but this quickly extends to working the upper half of the body and the lower half. We often see in a young baby the head, chest and arms reaching out and the lower half of the body working together to thrust back. This combination of actions is known as a *homologous* pattern. In the arch position of the Cat, the top half of the body moves in one direction as the bottom half moves in the other to recreate this sense of the homologous movement.

The next stage is the *homolateral* pattern: one side of the body moves together, right arm with right leg and left arm with left leg with the spine swivelling, rather like a lizard.

Movement from arched to rounded spine is led by the head.

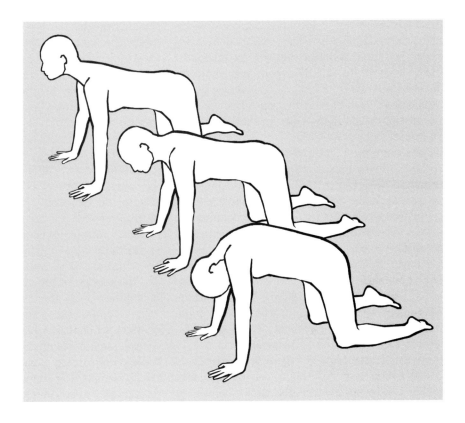

1. In the Cat position, turn the head to the right to bring your right foot into vision and then make the same action to the left side. As you do so, your shoulder and hip will come closer together in a *homolateral* action that really engages the upper back.
2. The final stage is the *contralateral* or *bilateral* pattern where opposite limbs work together. Take the Cat into a crawling action where right knee moves with left hand, and left knee with right hand.
3. This is repeated as we walk, swinging our left arm to counterbalance our right leg and right arm to counterbalance the left leg. Try this in action, being conscious of this cross-patterning.

As soon as we move out of childhood these even patterns of movement soon become distorted as we start to favour one side over the other and develop tensions in the body. We may be aware of our own *bilateral* imbalances as one hip may be tighter than the other (lie on the floor and see if your feet open out evenly). Moshe Feldenkrais understood that our physical limitations are self-imposed and that our repeated and habitual imbalances lead to a narrowing not just in our movements but in our entire functioning. His work explores some of these fundamental movement patterns and allows us to relay pathways to the nervous system and rediscover a more innocent body. You will discover that many of the qualities and principles we have identified in relation to the Alexander technique, could also be thought of as true for the Feldenkrais Method.

THE FELDENKRAIS METHOD

Together with the Alexander Technique, the Feldenkrais Method has proved itself the most influential holistic practice used by performers over the last fifty years. Many of the outcomes and concepts underlying Feldenkrais work are essentially rather similar to those employed in Alexander, but the ways of getting there are actually quite different. In fact, far from being contradictory, the two methods have a surprising amount in common. Each shares the belief that the individual must take responsibility for their own body by acknowledging bad habits and taking part in a holistic body–mind enterprise based on a spirit of enquiry. Championed by theatre visionary Peter Brook, the Feldenkrais Method is used extensively in actor training academies and amongst dance companies throughout the world, and continues to attract devotees especially in the field of physical theatre.

As we discovered in Chapter 1, in Alexander work the teacher's guiding hands encourage the pupil to undertake the everyday actions of sitting, walking, lying and standing in a more aligned and centred way, using touch and helpful visualizations to reconnect the body to its 'innocent' self. In the Feldenkrais Method, there is generally a different emphasis. Although teacher guidance sessions exist in Feldenkrais work, known as *Functional Integration*, they are often for those who have suffered injuries or traumas and have difficulty responding to direction. The usual method is a group lesson known as *Awareness Through Movement*. In an ATM lesson, you will find yourself lying on the floor, probably amongst a group of others, listening to a series of detailed directions from the teacher. As you listen to the teacher's guiding words, you slowly begin to respond, via a series of tiny movements, each repeated many times. Feldenkrais believed that changes to the tonus of the muscle would occur once the body had experienced the action about twenty-five times. Although he did not wish to be prescriptive about an exact number of times a movement should be executed, repetition is certainly a key feature of the Method, bringing with it inestimable improvements to kinaesthetic awareness. The clusters of repeated movements contribute to the development of a very finely tuned sensory perception that we probably haven't experienced since we were babies making discoveries about how to roll ourselves over and shift off the spot.

The tiny isolated movements unravel the muscles, loosen the joints and open up the senses in very surprising ways. Once you have experienced and understood the movement lessons in your own body, you are free to practise the movements by yourself, discovering increasingly deep levels of release. In the early stages it is far preferable to work under the guidance of an experienced teacher.

Each lesson pays attention to different parts of the body and how they relate to each other. As you practise the sequences of movements, you will often experience a sense of release as the body is liberated from tensions and habitual misuse. This experience can be immensely valuable for creative work. Ultimately, it can have a powerful effect on the capacity for physical expression. Moreover, in working with the Feldenkrais 'lessons', the whole organization of the body undergoes subtle changes, as our movement becomes increasingly refined and gradually recovers the 'innocence' experienced in early childhood. In time, and as a result of working mindfully with Feldenkrais movements, many students report being able to think more clearly and move both in and out of the performance space in a far more connected and focused way. Feldenkrais work is essentially an *experiential* method in which the student learns to tune in to internal changes in the body and regard the lessons as an adventure in recovering innocent movement. In Feldenkrais work, the journey from your back to sitting, or rolling from your back onto your front can take on the epic proportions of a journey in space. This can be compared to the Alexander experience of sitting to standing and back again that, when performed in an 'innocent' way, can feel momentous. These practices teach us to experience familiar actions in ways that our bodies have almost forgotten.

MOSHE FELDENKRAIS

Moshe Feldenkrais was a physicist who became particularly fascinated by the dynamics of the moving body. A black belt in judo, he began experimenting with his own patterns of use in order to try to alleviate physical ailments of his own. As a result of this work, he evolved a system for which he devised more than a thousand 'lessons' to help people acquire for themselves, a more efficient and graceful movement capacity. He worked not only with performers of all kinds, but also with children and people suffering from debilitating illnesses, including stroke victims. The Feldenkrais approach proved highly curative in helping the individual relearn muscle use, by stimulating parts of the brain that had become inert. Even in an apparently healthy person, said Feldenkrais, whole sections of the body can, over time, become dulled, unresponsive and ultimately lifeless. The method helps to stimulate these so-called 'dead' parts into a new sense of vitality and a fluent reconnection with the rest of the body.

Expanding the Self

The other effect of freeing up locked parts of the body by reorganising movement patterns, is that this work can greatly help the development of confidence. Feldenkrais believed that around the age of 13, many people have already made a decision in life about what they think they will or will not be capable of doing and at this time start to shut down all sorts of opportunities for themselves. It is no coincidence that this re-luctance to try things out occurs at the same time as the teenage body frequently begins to close off from the world and lose spontaneity. By using Feldenkrais work to release the body, those lost opportunities often return to the individual who will gain a sense of real empowerment by prac-tising the lessons. The innocent body is also a body full of promise.

Rather like Alexander, Feldenkrais saw the body as a metaphor for human potential and believed that if we could learn to recover lost function in the muscle, this would offer a person an expanding sense of themselves that could then be applied to all kinds of areas beyond the purely physical, For the performer, the method offers the chance to develop an extraordinary sensitivity in the body that can be harnessed in expressing character and/or in developing a highly refined movement vocabulary that can be brought into play in all sorts of performance contexts.

The following consists of a series of inter-connecting 'lessons' that can be explored as a cumulative sequence. Don't try to do them all in one go but build up slowly, working through from start to finish. Suggestions are offered for how you might integrate the breathing with the movement patterns but you don't have to be slavish about this. You will soon begin to experience what feels naturally right and it is important not to become so rigid about breathing that you actually lose the flow of the movements.

A Fundamental Feldenkrais Lesson – Bringing the Leg to 'Standing' with Minimal Effort

Allow plenty of time for Feldenkrais work. It works best if you take it really slowly.

Preparation

Lie on your back on a large mat or a couple of large soft blankets in a warm place. Wear loose, warm clothes and some thick socks. It's important to have a sense of security and comfort on the floor. It should feel a very safe and natural place to be.

1. Begin by lying down carefully stretching your legs out in front of you. Tune into your breathing and observe its passage. Be present and allow a moment of space between the full inhalation as it turns itself around into the exhalation and again, when the exhalation ceases, to allow the new breath to come in. See if it's possible to lengthen both the inhalation and the exhalation. Notice if one foot turns out more than another. This will tell you something about a possible bilateral imbalance in the body. One hip may be tighter than the other. Just observe this as a matter of interest but don't make any judgements.

2. Now, draw your legs up and arrive in semi-supine with your feet 'standing' on the mat beneath your knees, about hip-width apart. This happens also to be the classic Alexander *semi-supine* position; it is often used as a starting position in Feldenkrais work.

3. Notice the sensation of your back on the floor. What is happening here? Do the two sides of

the back feel even? Make sure your feet are placed to support your knees without excess muscular effort. They should be placed so that the legs will support themselves, not clamped together or in danger of falling apart. Experiment to discover what seems to be the best position for your feet in relation to your body, in which your legs can be self-supporting. Too far away and your legs may slide away from you. Too close and the knees will want to fall in or out.

4. Keep a sense of your right foot being connected to the ground though not by tensing it up. Inhale.

5. As you exhale, allow the left knee to open to the side and as it reaches its maximum, slowly slide the left foot away from you extending the leg towards the end of the mat in one continuous movement.

6. Reverse the action on an in breath, making sure that you pass the knee through the outward rotation, softly arriving at your starting position in semi-supine as you reach full inhalation. Keep the movement fluent.

7. Repeat six times with the left leg straightening down and back again and the right foot planted on the ground. Feel the connection between the 'standing' leg and the releasing leg. See what happens if you try the movement with a 'floppy' or unawake standing foot. You may find that the movement of the extending leg just collapses. Try again with a foot that *thinks itself* into the ground and you will discover a quite different quality of movement.

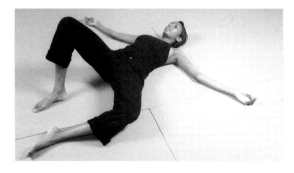

Leg lengthening to the ground on the out breath.

8. Now repeat the breath-led movements with the right leg keeping the left foot as your stable base.

When you have really got the feel of the movements and have learned to synchronize the actions (or 'actures' as Feldenkrais called them) with the breathing, you can try to shift from one leg to another as follows:

9. This time, as you bring the leg up through centre at the end of the inhalation, begin to shift the other leg down to the ground on the exhalation without making any break between alternate legs. This has the effect of allowing you to roll through the pelvis from side to side in one continuous action. You should feel quite free to roll through the back of the pelvis and sacrum as you shift through the movements from side to side. The most important thing is to keep the movements happening smoothly with the breath leading the rhythm.

10. Rest with your legs stretched out in front of you. Observe the position of your feet and see whether this has altered from your first observation in 1.

11. After this lesson, slowly get up and walk around. Feel what is happening in your lower body. You may feel more connected to the earth. A lot of people feel much wider and freer in their walking after experiencing this fundamental Feldenkrais sequence.

Playfulness and Flow

One of the hallmarks of the Feldenkrais Method, and a concept that lies at the heart of the *Innocent Body*, is that of *playfulness*. It is often pointed out that in Feldenkrais exercises we generally start on our backs. We are returned to the place where it all began, when as babies we launched ourselves into the world with our first tentative forays into the world around us. In Feldenkrais work, experimenting with small movements makes us curious to discover both the limits and the expansive possibilities of the body. In this, we are really only recovering sensations we all experienced as babies.

Knees resting in palms.

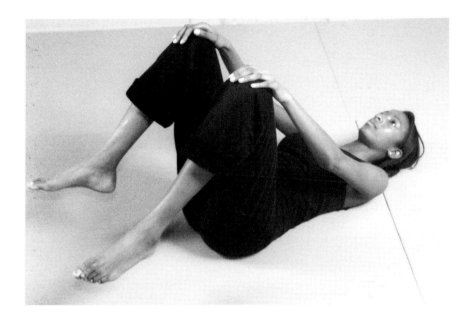

Very often, the repeated practice of a movement will take us unawares into quite another movement and this element of surprise is one of the unexpected delights of the work. For example, movements such as lying, sitting and standing that may have become awkward and disconnected in our adult bodies, in Feldenkrais work may suddenly begin to flow from one to another through fluent interconnecting movements. Feldenkrais practice restores this flow as the sharp corners and edges of adult movement are erased. In order for this to happen, we need to work with careful attention and to learn how to use only the essential muscles required for a given action. The idea is not to engage unnecessary peripheral muscle but only the actual joint or muscle group required. Think of how a centipede moves each individual segment of his length to caterpillar itself along – the ultimate in terms of isolating movement. The theatre director Stanislavski wrote about this ideal state for the performer, in a famous 'piano' metaphor. He recommended that the actor move not by crashing the body through discordant clumps of notes but learning to play each note separately, black as well as white. The result is a body that knows how to articulate itself with great accuracy, delicacy and economy. The Feldenkrais challenge is to differentiate only the essential muscles required for a movement and to make that movement as simple and clear as if sounding the *semitones* of the body. This is a body that can improvise playfully.

Finding the Body's Play

Try the following sequences but be careful not to cut corners. Give each set of movements its full time and space, respecting the rest periods. Remember babies do not have deadlines: the work is essentially explorative. The movements can be tiring especially if the body has been very stuck; it takes a while to recover after each round of 'actures'. The movements are cumulative and should be performed in sequence, with time in between to rest in semi-supine. You should even get up and walk around to feel the changes in the body and reflect on the freer sense of movement.

1. Begin by lying on your back as usual in semi-supine and performing the leg releasing exercise detailed above. Return to semi-supine and rest, feeling the changes in the body and the increased connection with the ground across the sacrum and the pelvis.
2. Now, begin the second sequence. From semi-supine, lift your feet off the ground. Hold your

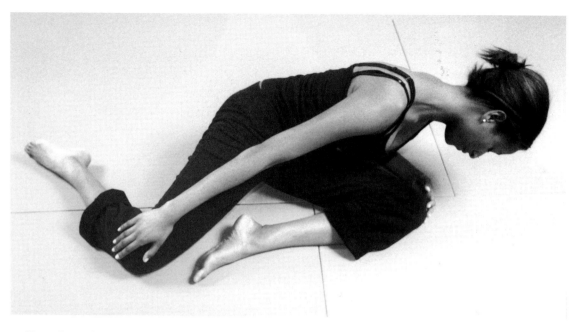

Rolling through from lying to sitting.

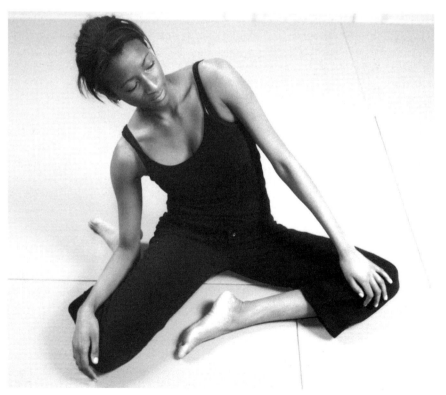

Arriving in sitting.

knees in the palms of your hands without tensing up and breathe well.

3. Inhale and allow the right hip to open by letting the right knee slowly descend towards the floor on the right as you exhale. Return to the centre on the inhalation and repeat.

4. Continue to perform the actions until you feel your weight roll to the right bringing the right knee towards the floor. On an exhalation, allow it to release down and at the last moment, let the left knee follow it downwards. Just before it arrives on top of the right knee, and still holding with the left palm, allow the left knee to move down and away towards your right foot, keeping parallel to the ground until the knee comes down to rest. As you experiment with this action, follow your left knee with your nose and this will help you to get flexion and roundness.

What happens to your torso when you put this movement into action?

5. Try the action a few times, carefully returning the legs to the centre on each inhalation. Let the breath do the movements. If you keep your head low to the ground as you exhale the leg to the floor and away from you, you may soon find that you are actually sitting!

6. Repeat this sequence, carefully passing through each stage of the movements up to twenty-five times on both sides to discover how easy and effortless this action can be.

7. Eventually, you will discover how to move from lying to sitting on one side and then returning through centre to sit on the opposite side. Try a few times, but remember this is tiring. Stop to rest whenever you need to. Return to semi-supine and note the changes in contact with the floor.

Developing Playfulness

1. For the next Feldenkrais sequence, lie on the floor again as before and observe the breathing once more. This time, lightly let the soles of your feet come together and your knees fall apart.

2. Either hold onto the outside edge of the feet with your hands or your big toes with your index fingers, whichever is more comfortable.

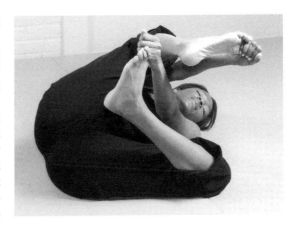

Developing playfulness.

3. Now, letting your feet come off the ground, play with the action of flexing the knees to the sides and then extending the legs alternately. Try letting one leg extend as the other foot moves in towards you, knee falling to the side.

4. Roll from side to side on your back through your hips and shoulders as you bend and extend from side to side. Try as before to synchronize the extending leg with the out breath and the inward-bound movement with the in breath. Recall the image of a baby with its foot in its mouth and see if you can get back into your own movements that sense of playful exploration. Imagine you are performing these movements for the first time, like the baby seeing just what your body is capable of. Roll from side to side, alternately extending and folding in your legs. Feel the movement through the hips.

5. Now, freely improvise your movements, sometimes allowing both legs to extend together and trying your elbows both outside and inside your bent legs.

Reorganizing the Shoulders and Spine

We store a great deal of tension in the shoulders and upper back. The following sequence is one of the many Feldenkrais lessons that help to reorganize this area, beginning with the impetus in the foot and allowing movement to travel through

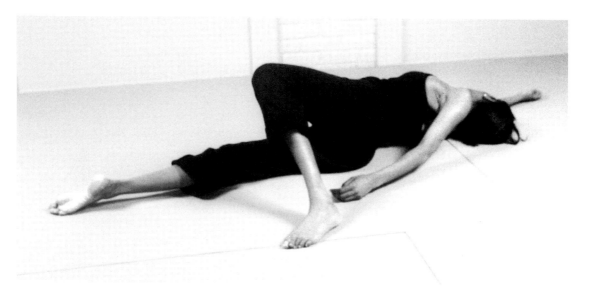

Reorganizing the shoulders and spine.

the bones of the body to the extended fingertips. This lesson builds on the very first Feldenkrais leg and hip reorganization lesson that we started off with and incorporates a reaching action of the arms and shoulders to create a whole-bodied movement.

1. Start on the back in semi-supine with the arms to the side of the body.
2. Scan the body, noting any areas of 'holding'. Follow the passage of your breath and observe any areas that seem resistant to the breath.
3. Revisit the leg and hip reorganization sequence detailed earlier in the chapter.
4. Once you have rediscovered the sensation of the leg and hip sequence, we will now develop the movement into a diagonal plane. Notice that when you press down with the heel of the right foot, the weight naturally rocks a little onto the opposite hip through the pelvis. Play with this cross-patterning movement, observing how the hip on the side where the foot is pressing wants to lift up and away from the ground.
5. Straighten the left leg as the right foot continues to press into the ground, so that the right hip can lift further, involving the spine

more and more. Return the left leg back to its starting position on the in breath.
6. Experiment with this pelvic rolling movement, many times, keeping contact with the floor through the right foot. The movement will be clearer if the right knee stays above the right ankle. Slowly come to standing and walk around feeling the difference in the right and left side.
7. Repeat the movement of pressing the right foot into the ground, and rolling the pelvis, as you extend the left arm over the head on the floor above and behind you. Feel the relationship of the right foot and the left arm through the spine and sense how these actions are connected. As you extend the left arm, the left leg will naturally want to lengthen to the ground. As the movement develops the turning head may naturally leave the floor as you turn to look at the outstretched arm.
8. With the inhalation, return to centre bringing in the left leg and arm. As you continue these movements, you may feel the impulse to lift the head as the spine arches further. See how the action of connecting the eyes with the reaching helps the movement and allows the action to occur more naturally. Practise this

action many times until it becomes clear and comfortable.

9. Always maintain the sense that the right foot is connected to the floor and initiates the movement.

10. Return to the centre and rest on your back allowing some time to reflect on the changes. Walk and observe changes.

11. Repeat the entire sequence on the other side, making sure you pass through all the movements and are not tempted to short-cut.

Teddy Bear Rolls

When you feel at ease with the previous sequences, you can experiment with some exhilarating *teddy bear rolls* that link all the other movements together in a continuous circular action. You may well have performed these movements for fun as a child.

You will need a large matted or carpeted area to work on. Slowly develop the sequence as this will allow for an improved quality of movement.

1. Begin in the starting position for the Developing Playfulness sequence, sitting up and holding the big toes.

2. Now, roll over to the right side and instead of rocking back to centre try to continue the roll in a big circle coming up to sitting and return to lying again by rolling down onto the left hip.

3. The important thing is not to end-gain and anticipate where the movement is taking you, but to stay in the movements from moment to moment, remembering to keep the nose close to the knee as you come up and go down again. You will feel yourself passing through many of the movements you have already done in order to prepare for this rolling action.

4. Try rolling in a continuous direction in big circles and then see if you can change direction. Really allow yourself to sense the movement through the entire pelvic and shoulder girdles, which glide across the surface of the floor.

Some people will remember quite quickly the joys of teddy bear rolling and they will soon be rolling

around in a stage of elation. For others, there may be initial frustration. Don't tighten up. The movements that both feel and work best are light and fluent, performed without effort or strain. Keep trying the preliminary movements, and it will suddenly happen.

Encouraging Awareness by Colouring the Bones

We have spoken a lot so far about the concept of awareness in relation to holistic practices. One of the ways in which Feldenkrais tried to awaken mind/body awareness is through what we could call a form of *experiential anatomy* in which the individual is taken on a kind of tour of the internal landscape of the body. This happens when the Feldenkrais teacher gives us directions to *colour the bones* with an imaginary paintbrush. The effect of this kind of lesson is that the skeletal bones become increasingly real, less mysterious and more *present* to us. It's interesting how this simple activity of the mind in relation to the body causes us to feel our

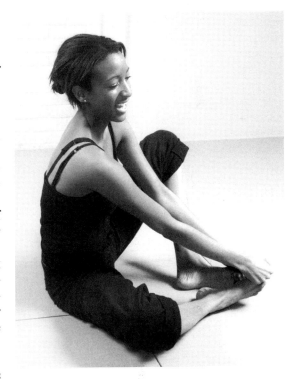

Preparing to teddy bear roll.

bones in a different way. As we begin to trust our bones to take the weight and momentum of our moving body, unwelcome muscle tension loses its grip, we feel our skeletons more clearly and so are more able to use them in an articulate way. As we get a better sense of how this all happens, we can learn to let go of unnecessary tensions which, in turn, frees breath and movement. Performers could try this exercise with specific colours relating to character or mood. Keep the colour consistent as you paint the whole body.

What Can Be Done?

All this sounds quite negative. However, both practitioners were evangelical in the belief that something could be done by developing the right outlook. In their separate and individual ways, both Feldenkrais and Alexander believed that if the individual took responsibility for their own mind/ body wellbeing, many of the damaging effects of misusing the body could be remedied. At the heart of this was the notion that an individual should *actively* engage in the work rather than passively expecting someone else to do it for them. Even in Alexander work, which is apparently dependent on a teacher, there is an expectation that the 'pupil' will respond kinaesthetically and endeavour to put the principles into action in daily living. Both practices regard the development of mind–body awareness as a journey of learning that is never completed; as such, those receiving instruction are nearly always referred to as pupils or students rather than clients.

According to these two visionaries, it is far more useful to be engaged in the idea of process rather than product (Alexander called this *the means whereby* we do something as opposed to *end-gaining*). Concentrating on how we do something rather than giving too much attention to what we are aiming for, avoids the damaging habit of straining after results that can so easily make the body tense up. Being open and interested in the idea of a journey of exploration makes us far softer, more open and spontaneous.

By consciously using either or both of these bodywork practices, a performer can increase their physical *awareness* to the point where they will

---

Links Between the Feldenkrais Method and Alexander Technique

Although, as we have seen, the practices are quite different, both Feldenkrais and Alexander shared some common thinking, including the belief that as we grow older we frequently damage ourselves through misusing our bodies in the following ways:

- we waste vast amounts of energy by holding unnecessary tensions in our body;
- we often use far more muscular effort to perform simple actions than we need;
- our bodies get locked into bad habits such as slouching or holding ourselves unevenly, which in the course of time exert a negative effect on our whole being;
- our fear of failure often causes us to hold our breath or breathe shallowly and this reduces our energy;
- muscles become short and tight losing their ability to spiral;
- we forget to 'listen' to our own bodies;
- we lose a sense of grace, ease and 'innocence'.

---

benefit from long-lasting and meaningful changes both in body and in attitude. For these approaches, an openness to new ways of learning leading to the possibility of *change* is the most important element. Very often this involves the abandonment of fixed patterns and habits that have long encrusted the body. Engaging in Alexander work or the Feldenkrais Method can feel like shedding an old skin and discovering underneath something far more innocent and vulnerable than our old deadlocked selves. In this way, by working sensitively to experience solutions to physical challenges, and resisting the seduction of old ways of being, it's possible to develop the capacity for originality that has enormous implications for the creative process. This work does require risk and investment, not just on a physical level but also an emotional level, in order to open up the capacity for creativity.

3 YIN AND YANG

THE INFLUENCE OF YIN/YANG-RELATED PRACTICE ON WESTERN PERFORMANCE

In the west over the last fifty years, physical philosophies deriving from Asia have been immensely significant to the development of performance-related bodywork. The concept of *yin and yang* lies at the heart of many disciplines ranging from martial arts to healing therapies that performers have tapped into for the discovery and release of vital stores of energy, balance and wellbeing. An awareness of the qualities of yin/yang even underpins western holistic movement forms like Contact Improvisation (*see* Chapter 5) that grew out of Steve Paxton's interest in aikido, and the Feldenkrais Method (*see* Chapter 2) that wouldn't have been developed without Moshe Feldenkrais's formative experience of judo. This chapter explores yin and yang in relation to tai chi, Chinese stick work and shiatsu.

EAST AND WEST – DIFFERENT WAYS OF VIEWING HUMANS IN RELATION TO NATURAL FORCES

Central to eastern philosophies of the body is the fundamental link between human beings and the universe. In eastern thinking, human life is part of the greater cosmic pattern, with forces deriving from the five *transformations* or *elements* (in Taoist thinking these are earth, water, fire, wood, metal). Characteristics of human behaviour and physicality are likened to forces and states that already exist in nature. This idea differs from the prevailing belief in western cultures by which humans are seen almost to be superior to nature rather than a reflection of nature. In the west, for hundreds

of years now, and certainly since the Age of Reason, the human mind has been privileged over the body and the natural universe, and rational thinking, especially scientific thinking, prized above all else. The body (a manifestation of *nature* as opposed to *reason*) has been thought of as a machine that can be driven by the mind and fixed if it breaks down. The body and mind in western thinking have been considered as separate entities, an opposition in which the mind is regarded as superior to the body. This kind of dualism is a characteristic of capitalist cultures in which, in very simplistic terms, competition and achievement are highly valued. In the west, the activity of *doing* (yang/active) is often regarded as more important than *being* (yin/passive). In the east however, the yin/yang pairing is not thought of in terms of opposing but as complementary forces working together.

THE NATURE OF YIN AND YANG

The concept of yin and yang is a way of looking at the world that is about identifying and relating to complementary forms of energy, both within us and outside us. According to yin/yang theory there are no absolutes. Instead, forms are considered to be yin or yang in relation to one another depending on which one is 'more so': they represent a continuum as one transforms into another. The following sets of pairings may give an idea of classic yin/yang properties but these can alter depending on the comparison; so for example water is *yin* in relation to steam, but *yang* in relation to ice.

- *Yin:* gravity and earth, moon, night, dark, maturity, storing up energy through being, cool, contracting, inhalation.

- *Yang:* rising up and heavenward, sun, day, light, youth, releasing energy through doing, hot, expanding, exhalation.

Yin is like the ovum and yang is like the sperm. Therefore yin is sometimes thought of as female and yang as male, although it is simplistic to suggest masculine/feminine characteristics are always gender specific. Many men have strong yin characteristics (reflective, observant) and women can be predominantly yang (dynamic, outgoing) in temperament. Neither yin nor yang ever remains in one state indefinitely, but will always be subtly shifting and transforming to its opposite condition.

Yin and Yang Symbol – Tai Ji

Look at the symbol to see how the two sides are not separated like two halves but are curled around one another, leaning on one another.

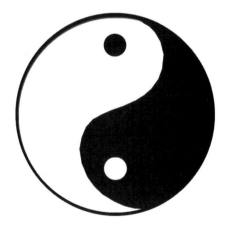

Tai Ji – the Yin Yang symbol.

You may notice that each side has a little dot of the opposite colour in its centre. This symbolizes the idea that there is always some yin in the yang and some yang in the yin – they are never completely separate because they contain their opposite. Just as the cosmos needs both the sun and moon, each of us have both yin and yang within us – we are neither wholly one thing nor the other but need to find a dynamic balance. So, in performance there is never a fixed state, but one that is organic and evolving. One of the crucial ideas behind yin/yang

theory is the concept that the quality of the energy is forever shifting and changing, never static. The way to think about the symbol is not to visualize it as a fixed image but liken it more to the symbol of a white fish and a black fish mating, forever in motion. This thought captures the spirit of the constant vitality of the yin/yang interchange, the amoeba-like shape that represents constant flow.

The Yin/Yang Fish

The following exercise is a way of embodying the symbol and flowing with the yin-yang exchange.

1. In pairs, stand opposite one another.
   Shake your right hands and then take each other's right elbows with the other hand so that you make a circle resembling the yin/yang fish. Keep flexible wrists, elbows and hips and begin to play with shifting the fish around in the constantly moving circle of water you have created.
2. Keep knees and neck soft and practise sympathetic breathing (breathing in tune with your partner) from your stomach centre as you duck and weave with the yin/yang fish. Your arms, shoulders and whole body will feel more mobile and energized as you give and take weight and space. The circle of energy is created through the confluence of yin/yang spiralling.

Yin/Yang in Performance
Yin and yang in the performance context can exist in at least four different ways:

- The performer's awareness of their own energy qualities.
- The performer's understanding of the energy qualities required by their role or score.
- The exchange of energy between performers onstage.
- The exchange of energy between performer and audience.

Predominantly yang-type active people often have to learn to conserve their strength and develop a more reflective aspect whereas those who tend to be more yin, have to find the impetus to push themselves into action through discovering a more dynamic form of expression. Obviously this inclination towards one or the other energy quality can alter from moment to moment during the day as our moods and energy levels shift. What can go wrong is when the yin/yang tendencies are habitually out of balance, which can result in either burnout or lethargy. In theatrical terms this imbalance can manifest itself in a performance that is either unremittingly forceful or too introspective and hidden. Any dialogue, whether it's spoken, physical or musical – between performers themselves or performance and an audience – requires the forces of yin and yang to be in a state of *fluidity*. The performer has to be acutely aware that s/he is the conduit for this exchange and be capable of subtly transforming it. Although one associates theatrical performance with being very *yang* (out there), to be effective it needs to have at its core a very yin quality of focus and sensitivity. Physical theatre has formed its identity around being vibrant and hyper-energetic. It's dependent on a very yang-like quality, that can at worst appear forceful and aggressive (in yer face). However, if tempered with moments of stillness or lyricism, when the yang quality has yin at its centre, it becomes far more powerful. An example would be the famous production of Macbeth by the Japanese director Ninagawa, in which scenes of violence and murder were played to the backdrop of lyrical music and exquisite falling petals. The sole expression of either yin or yang can be flat and dreary without the opposite force providing a contrasting tension. When there is a successful performance moment, the qualities of yin and yang never exist in isolation but are counterpointed. This is the case, whether contained in the entire stage picture or in the single performance. So, for example, a contemplative moment should always contain a sense of strength and inner dynamism and a dynamic moment will have a quality of inner stillness.

Finding the Sensation of Yin and Yang in the Body – Sun and Moon Breathing

This is a simple four-way exercise to feel the qualities of yin and yang energies in the body. This

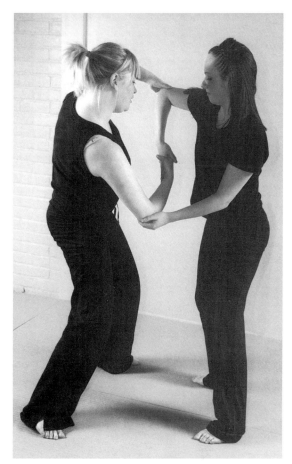

The yin/yang fish.

cycle of yin inhalation and yang exhalation represents the waxing and waning of the sun and moon. Initially, it may help to actually sound the breathe as you breath in and out listening for the difference in energy quality. It is important to relax the neck and feel the ground so that when you lift the arms, the shoulders remain lowered and do not start to move toward the ears.

1. On the in breath, raise the arms to the side of the body until they are level with the shoulders. Think of gathering in the fresh air with a sense of gentle surrender as you soften the knees (YIN).

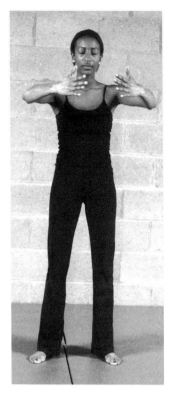
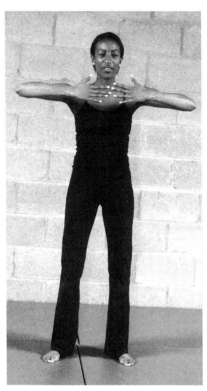
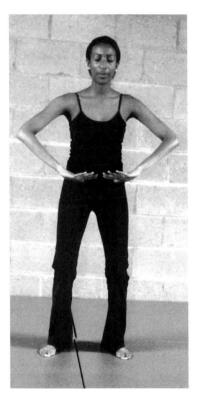

Yang breath, pushing forward.

Yin breath, gathering in.

Yang breath, pushing down.

2. On the out breath thrust the arms forward and together, with a sense of power and resistance, until the palms face one another keeping them in line with the shoulders. Think of pushing out the stale air on a sustained out breath as you allow the legs to straighten (YANG).

3. As you breathe in, bring the palms forward towards the chest softly gathering in the air once more and allowing the knees to release as you make the inward movement (YIN).

4. On the out breath push the palms downward towards the floor strongly, as you lengthen the spine and straighten the legs, stretching the body up towards heaven and the hands down towards earth (YANG).

Repeat the sequence several times, deepening your connection with the flow of yin and yang.

Finding the Yang Energy – the Executioner's Chop

This is an effective exercise to generate a strong sense of yang if feeling sluggish or needing to summon powerful energy. In performance the actor or musician may have to produce a sudden moment of intense passion or even anger, which is about harnessing and releasing an inner power. This exercise can help you tap into that force. It may help if you accompany the movements with a specific motivation. Some people find it difficult to produce aggression and for them it's helpful instead to think in terms of protecting or defending something or someone very precious.

1. Stand with feet apart and body centred as if in the shape of an A. Breathe with arms outstretched and palms together.

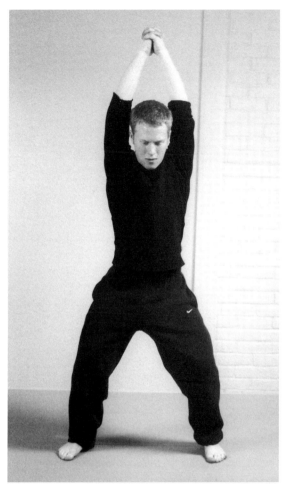

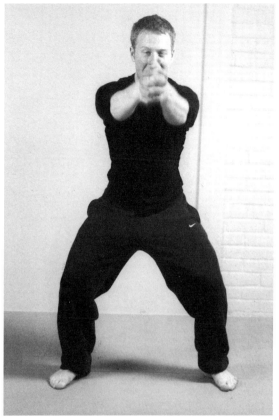

LEFT: *Executioner's chop 1.*

ABOVE: *Executioner's chop 2.*

2. As you inhale, slowly raise your arms up through your centre taking three steps in front of you and centring your weight as you walk. On the fourth step, return to the A stance. Time the steps, the arms and the breath so you are at your maximum inhalation as you take the fourth step that brings your feet back to parallel, reaching the highest point with your arms.

3. Look down and gather yourself in this moment of transition between the in breath and the out breath.

4. Forcefully slash your arms down through your centre, simultaneously raising your head as you emit a sharp 'ha' of sound on the out breath.

Spring to Action

Another yang-raising activity is to start in the upright kneeling position (with the toes and the knees sharing in supporting the weight of the body). Take a deep breath in, and on the outbreath, drawing energy from your lower abdomen, leap into the air and land in a squat position. This feels like a really challenging exercise but it's amazing how the power of the explosion will generate the movement. It is particularly powerful when done in a group.

Finding the Yin Energy – Butoh Walk

Sometimes the most compelling character on stage can be the least vocal and active one. They may generate a mesmerizing intensity. The following

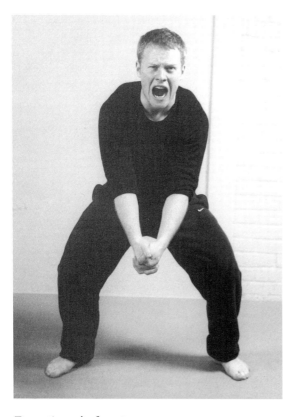

Executioner's chop 3.

exercise helps you discover that less is more. *Butoh* is a form of contemporary Japanese dance theatre that was created as a healing theatrical experience. In this style of performance, all action is distilled to elemental movements often performed at an excruciatingly slow pace. The Butoh walk is a challenging exercise that helps intensify and purify the performer's presence. Atmospheric music can enrich the following experiences.

1. Set a pathway of about 20 metres and walk along as slowly as you possibly can. The concentration will make you aware of your breathing.
2. Walk with a rolling movement shifting the weight from one foot through the pelvis to the other foot and keep the knees soft. You should experience the anatomy of walking in a very intense way.

3. Head must remain in a straight line with the neck free so that it becomes a glide. Allow the breath to flow freely.
4. The act of walking becomes primordial making you aware of the importance of stillness and the Zen principle of *being not doing*.

An extension of this exercise is to travel between two walls at as slow a pace as you possibly can, avoiding walking.

1. Start on your back and close your eyes. Slowly begin to shift yourself towards the opposite wall using gentle rolling, writhing or crawling movements originating from the abdomen.
2. Think of the evolutionary journey of the earliest sea creatures from the water to the land, or the birthing process, and be attentive to the blood and oxygen pumping the life-force within.

Heaven and Earth
As we have noticed, yang energy is directed upwards towards heaven whereas yin energy moves downwards towards the earth. Many of the exercises we have encountered help us to feel the connection with the ground. This was something that was observed by Alexander who was trying to tackle the western preoccupation with end-gaining and not being grounded and in the moment. Many Asian practitioners have noted the Western tendency to be very head-centred, whereas in the east the centre of being is the belly or the Hara in Japanese.

The Hara and the Dan Tien
The *hara* is the vital area where many of our organs are located and where yin (connected to the earth) meets yang (reaching to the sky). More specifically, the area about three fingers below the navel, deep inside the belly, is the spot known as the *dan tien* or *tant'ien*. For many Asian practices it is the fundamental centre of our movement, breath and being. This place is not only the physical centre but also the central repository of energy and the place from which the yin and yang are nurtured. Being physically mindful of this area allows all our

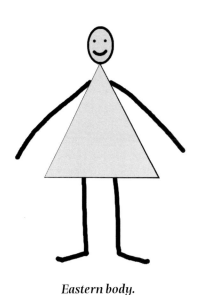

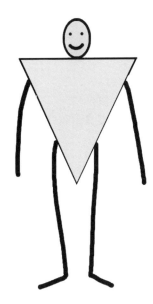

Eastern body.

Western body.

movements and actions to flow. In martial arts, including tai chi, the origin and inspiration of the movement comes from this point and returns to it. The arrangement of the hands in the classic meditation pose also draws energy and attention into this crucial centre. Media images in Western culture often highlight the chest (in both men and women) and the stomach is made to appear flat and invisible. Notice how this body ideal contrasts with images of Buddha where the fat stomach is seen to represent wisdom.

Sumo Swagger

One way to help feel connected with our hara is to adopt the position of the sumo wrestler before he launches into battle. Place the hands on the thighs with fingers pointing inwards and assume a semi-squat with knees apart. Now take a step forward keeping your hands on the thighs and as you do so make a strong grunting sound 'ha'! As you move forward, feel your body weight sinking into your hara and connecting with the ground beneath. Having activated this area (yang), take a few moments to place your hands at your dan tien, close your eyes and just breathe into this centre (yin).

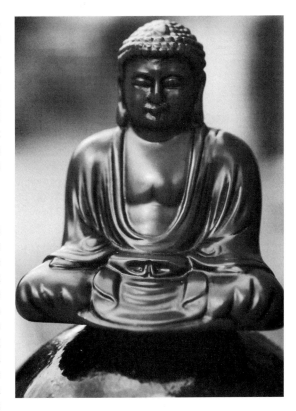

Buddha in classic meditation pose.

Now that you feel more connected to the hara, the practice of martial arts will become much more effective since you will have discovered the centre from which and to which all movements return.

TAI CHI – THE YIN/YANG DANCE

Tai Chi

- Developed originally in China by travelling monks around the twelfth century and now practised widely throughout the West.
- Tai Chi is known as a 'soft' martial art as opposed to aggressively 'hard' forms like Karate.
- Operates on the principle that rather than offering a yang opposition to attack, it is more effective to develop the art of softly yielding to force and recovering one's centre by means of curving back up again. (An activity known as 'Pushing Hands' develops this capacity by playing with the yin/yang forces in pairs – *see* Chapter 5).
- Involves a physical balancing and centering based on the spiralling action.
- Often practised outdoors placing great emphasis on responsiveness to the environment through listening with all the senses.
- Many styles of 'Tai Chi' are enormously complicated and place great emphasis on perfecting the form but the sequence we introduce is essentially playful with the emphasis on feeling the movement.
- Movements are often symbolic (like The Five Elements) – the form then becomes a kind of movement meditation.

Tai Chi Movement and the Curve

In the work we did earlier with Alexander and Feldenkrais, we learned the value of allowing a sense of spiralling in our body movement, reflecting the way the muscles wrap around the bones. These holistic techniques persuade us that the body is not just a series of parallel lines but is at its most graceful when we permit this gentle principle of unfolding to occur in our everyday movement. In Tai Chi work, the concept of the curve, the natural rotation and return to centre of the moving body, lies at the centre of the practice. There are no hard lines as there are none in nature itself. Just as we can think of the breath as being an enormous spherical balloon that gently inflates and deflates, so too should our tai chi movement, coming from below the navel at our centre (known as the *tant'ien* in tai chi), develop this quality of the sphere that rises and returns. As we send out energy on our movement, we gather it back in again to our centre. The curve that we send out always comes back to us, in a gentle boomerang action, and is essentially an expression of the yin/yang energy dyad.

The Yin-Yang Exchange – Stick Work

The idea of yin and yang relates to the notion of forces of *give and take*, of gathering up and releasing. This is a central consideration in the sphere of performance. At any given moment, there will be an interplay of all these forces at work and a good performer does not simply act on automatic pilot, but is both receptive (yin) and responsive (yang) to the changing energies around him/her, both on and off stage. Understanding what this exchange of energy is all about, and how to handle it, can be nurtured by an experience of yin/yang energy through stick work, used previously in the Chinese circus and the martial arts.

Partner Stick Work

Work in pairs. Keeping soft joints, apply the tai chi principle of responding to yang energy with a yielding yet playful strength.

Two lengths of bamboo sticks are required, around a metre in length. Atmospheric music with an interplay of lyrical/strong (yin/yang) rhythms.

1. Stand opposite your partner far enough away to balance a stick between your two sets of fingertips, a comfortable distance in front of you at about head height. Very slowly begin to move the sticks between you, feeling the

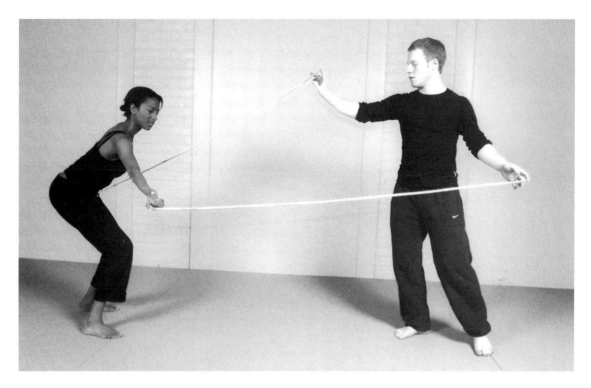

Stick work.

connection and being sensitive to your partner's impulse to move as well as your own. Resist the temptation to end-gain. You need to allow the movement into the whole body by loosening the hips and softening the knees. Don't forget to free the neck.

2. If you are both too yang you will be fighting for control, if you are both too yin, you will lose the connection and the sticks will probably drop. Don't be deterred, just pick them up and continue trying to balance the forces to sustain the flow. Keep taking it very slowly and feel your body releasing into the activity rather than holding on.

3. Keeping the sticks in contact, walk around. Be playful and take risks by climbing through the sticks and even moving onto the floor. Beware though, this is challenging for your focus of attention. Don't forget to breathe freely or you will lose the connection with your partner's energy. When the energy is balanced you will

feel as though you are touching fingertips directly. Remain slow.

4. Now close your eyes and enjoy experiencing the yin/yang flow through your fingertips using your kinaesthetic sense to guide you.

Once you have enjoyed the sensitivity of working in pairs, stick exercises work very effectively to build up an ensemble feeling. Try passing sticks in a circle keeping the rhythm steady and the sticks even. Then keep the sticks held still while bodies move around the circle.

The Five Elements: Earth, Water, Fire, Wood and Metal

Five Element (or Transformation) theory derives from *Traditional Chinese Medicine* and is an extension of the idea of yin/yang. Like yin/yang, it provides a means of thinking about some of the fundamental essences from which each human is constituted. Naturally, everyone is a mixture of

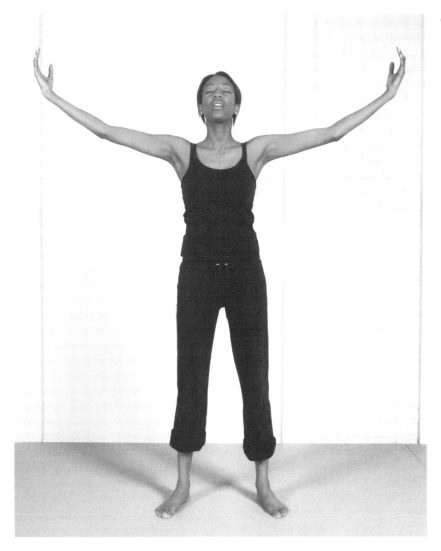

Opening from Earth.

these five qualities and the balance of this mixture will change from moment to moment as well as over time. However, if left to our own devices, we generally gravitate to one or more of these qualities of being that could be said to be 'our element'. So then, one person may be considered to be 'in their element' when planning and experiencing challenging new situations (Wood element), whereas another person may be 'in their element' in the safety and security of home (Earth element). A third person may be very emotional, spontaneous and creative (Fire element) a fourth

may be meticulous and organized (Metal element) and a fifth a fearful but often 'driven' person (Water element). Understanding how our individual constitutions relate to these classifications can help us know ourselves more thoroughly and to develop some of the elements within which we feel less familiar or comfortable. Performance often demands a comprehensive repertoire of behavioural types and tendencies and the ability to shift fluently from one state of being to another. This capacity can be developed through engaging in Five Element bodywork and feeling the resonance of the various elements in a whole-bodied, sensory, rather than abstract way. The Five Element Tai Chi sequence is a revealing starting place to begin this work.

Tai Chi Five Elements Sequence

This sequence, developed by the tai chi master Chungliang Al Huang from traditional tai chi movements, provides a way of physically experiencing the Five Elements. It allows the participant to come into contact with the essence of the elements. Every time you perform the Five Elements sequence you discover different responses depending on what is happening in your life. This experience can tell us a lot about our psycho-physical whereabouts. It is also a valuable exercise to perform in role and as it helps us to make some *somatic* responses to character. It is performed as a continuous sequence and begins and ends with the Earth element.

Earth

1. Legs need to be firmly grounded. Standing with legs in A stance, check that your knees are soft and drop the pelvis a little further towards the ground. Begin to breathe in as you bring the arms wide and up above the head finally allowing the tips of the fingers to touch together. The moment that the fingertips touch is a very exciting moment of transformation. As you reach upwards the legs will begin to straighten and you may have a sensation of opening into light and life.

2. Let the hands part like a bud bursting open. Bring them out and down to the side, descending in the same path as they ascended. As you bring them down, exhale, and let the knees soften down.

3. Again, sink down fractionally more with the legs as you once more begin to inhale. On the inhalation, the backs of hands now come up through the centre, past the tant'ien, grazing the front of the body to bring awareness of how self connects to the world beyond us

   As the hands reach the top above your head, so the legs straighten and then the arms burst open wide up again, falling as you exhale.

4. Let hands dangle as you now bring the forearms up to waist height, at which point you allow the wrists to float up and down once to come to rest, being at peace and security in the place of the mother earth.

Water

1. Take a step back onto your right foot and begin to enjoy a sense of shifting your weight through your base from foot to foot letting your arms flow out to balance and support the movement. This Element feels like a surfing movement as you bend, duck and dive, letting your centre and your upper limbs and head float and reel on the shifting momentum of your feet. It's as if you had water beneath your feet coming in huge unpredictable waves and bellows, which can be quite frightening but also exhilarating if you go with the flow.

2. As you feel the surges and tugs of this movement, it's as if you are turning and experiencing the world from all angles, your spine rotating freely whilst balancing over your tant'ien. This element is about adaptability so think soft joints, liquid body.

3. Envisage the depth of water beneath your feet and focus on your trust in the element and your ability to ride out the unexpected whilst keeping your peaceful centre.

Fire

1. From water, lift the back right foot up as you breathe in and then step on the foot pushing yourself forwards into the fire element with an exhalation. As you thrust the foot downwards, push the arms powerfully downwards through the centre and then upwards above and in ront of you. The sensation here is of suddenly igniting like flame bursting upwards. This movement is about danger, passion and exhilaration. The weight is now on the front foot.

2. As you inhale after your big fire out-breath, return the right foot to its place by the left as you draw the bodyweight back. In this parallel position, bring your arms down over your face and torso, with your fingertips gently sprink-

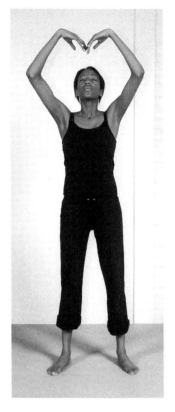

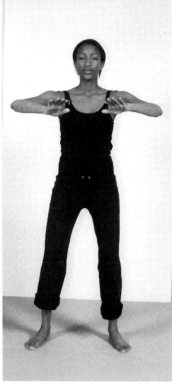

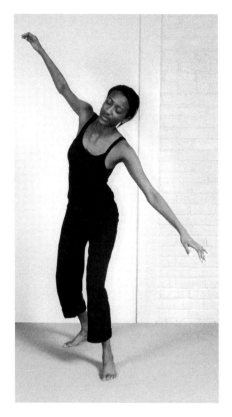

Coming up through the centre.

Return to Earth.

Surfing through water.

ling water all over the body, refreshing and cooling it after the heat of the fire back to the earth centre.

Wood

1. From this calm, centred position, begin to rotate the body to the left as far as you can, in a journey of exploration, stepping around when necessary to reach 180 degrees behind you. Embrace the adventure by using your eyes to explore all around you and taking your arms wide.

2. Then begin the journey back to the centre, having a sense of passing through the earth or home element but this time continue to tep around away from the centre, turning a full circle to bring you back finally to face the front.

The Wood element represents the journey of discovery as you move away from home and safety to face new challenges and risk. It's the element of adventure and growth.

Metal

1. Back at the earth centre, the right arm now reaches behind the body allowing the whole body from the ankles upwards to rotate behind you as far as you can without disturbing your stance. From this position, you pick up a 'treasure' that you then bring back to tant'ien.

2. Rotate now to the left as the left arm reaches behind to gather 'treasure' from the space behind the body and bring it forward into the tant'ien. It's a feeling of selecting something valuable and special that you have witnessed or experienced.

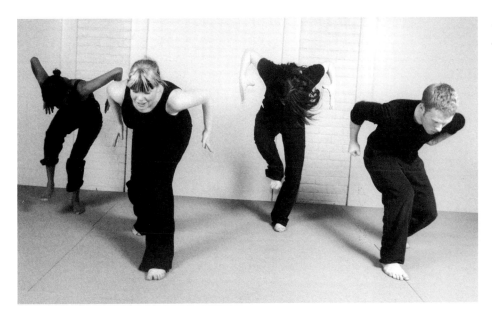

*Enter the
fire.*

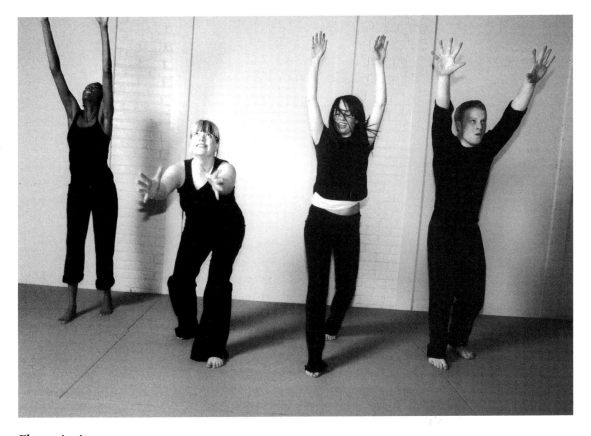

Flames ignite.

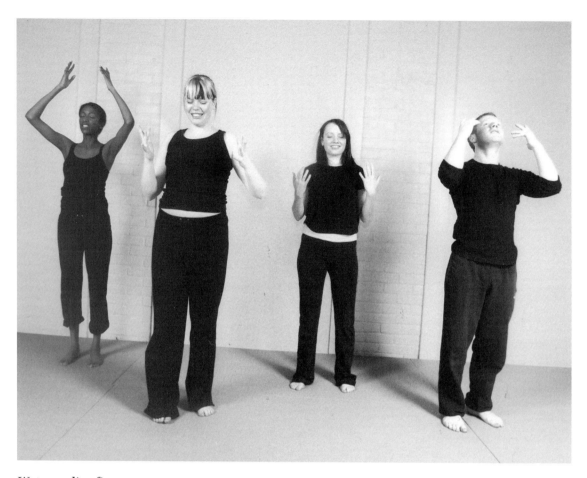

Water cooling fire.

3. Gather together and mix these treasures without touching hands, returning them to your own energy source in your tant'ien.

The metal element is about sorting, selecting and refining the experiences or your journeying and mixing them into new forms. It's a kind of alchemy relating to the creative process, which is about distilling and transforming experiences from our life journey. Now this journey is over, you can return to Earth. The whole sequence can now be repeated, taking the movements to the opposite side of the body from which you have just experienced them (that is, begin Water movements to left side, and so on).

Connecting with the Movements

The Five Elements sequence is essentially about feeling your relationship to the movements and not being too worried about making the perfect form. The important thing is to enjoy the movements by being really present so that you can then intuit your responses. You may be more attracted to the movement of one element over the others. Some are more yang and some more yin, and you may pick this up as you do the movement. The elements flow into one another and this is echoed in their relationship to the cycles and rhythms of our nature. You can see clearly the association with the seasons: spring represents new growth which is wood; summer is the hottest, most yang month

Wood journey.

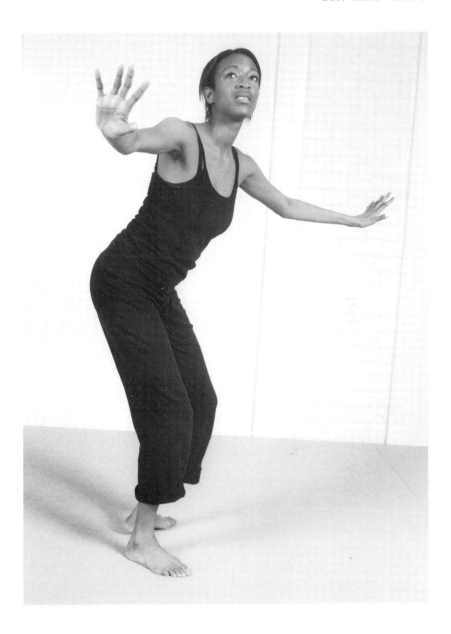

which is fire; late summer is the time for harvest, which is earth; autumn/fall is the time for nature to die down which is metal; and winter is water, the time for hibernation and storing of energy, which is the most yin of seasons. The elements are also associated with particular times of the day and colours, smells and sounds that invoke their quality. Look at the table on page 65 that gives a number of these properties.

The Performer and the Elements

You may immediately begin to relate to one or more of these elements. We are all likely to be a mixture of these, although at times one aspect may be dominant. An awareness of the personality tendencies can be particularly helpful for performers. You could say that in a group rehearsal the one with the ideas is fire, the one supporting and holding the centre is earth, the one organizing

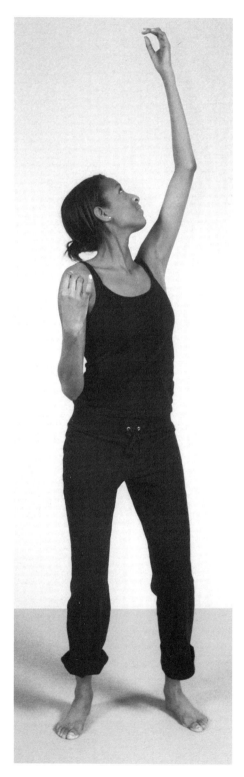

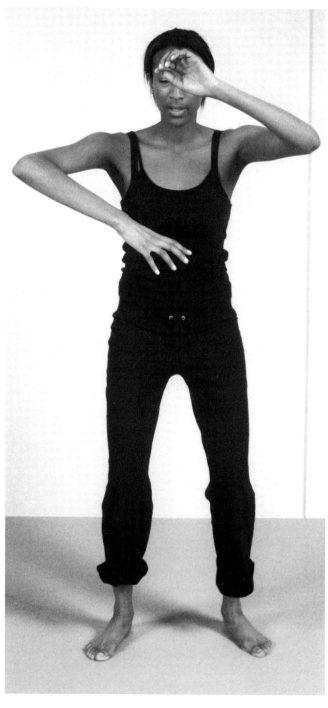

ABOVE: *Mixing the alchemy of the elements.*

LEFT: *Gathering metal treasure.*

Element	Meridian	Key Words	Personality Tendencies	Season	Senses and Body Parts	Emotions
Wood	Liver (yin) Gall bladder (yang)	Storage and plannning	Risk taking Initiating Leading Decisive	Spring	Eyes Muscles Tendons Ligaments	Anger
Fire	Heart (yin) Small Intestine (yang)	Interpretation and assimilation	Passionate Spontaneous Expressive	Summer	Tongue Blood vessels	Joy
Supplemental Fire	Triple Heater (yin) Heart constrictor (yang)	Protection and circulation	Absorbing and coping with strong emotions	Summer	Vascular and lymphatic systems	Joy
Earth	Spleen (yin) Stomach (yang)	Reproduction and digestion	Nurturing Caring Generous and stable	Late Summer	Mouth Flesh	Sympathy /worry
Metal	Lungs (yin) Large intestine (yang)	Exchange with the environment and elimination	Organizing Disciplined Appreciates order and beauty	Autumn	Nose Skin, body hair	Grief
Water	Kidneys (yin) Bladder (yang)	Purification and impetus	Articulate, Intelligent Surviving through adapting	Winter	Ears, Adrenals, Bones, Marrow	Fear

Five Elements Correspondences.

the schedule and editing material is metal, the one leading the session is wood and the one who questions and philosophizes is the water element. Try to think of people you know or even famous people who exemplify these elemental tendencies.

The Five Elements and the Meridians
The five elements contain a pair of meridian lines of Chinese Traditional Medicine; the only exception to this is Fire that has a supplementary pair. Each pair consists of a yin and yang meridian balancing the element. These meridians are pathways of energy that may not be visible but that are palpable beneath the skin. The meridians are linked to organs and functions of the body and

have both a physical and psychological dimension. They begin in the hara and radiate throughout the body. The diagrams shown in the next chapter give an indication of the key areas of the meridian lines used both by acupuncture and shiatsu practitioners.

If the energy of a meridian is out of balance this can result in either a depleted or an excessive state. The purpose of the shiatsu or acupuncture treatment is to restore harmony using an element or meridian to rebalance another.

Example of Element Imbalance
The earth element (stomach, spleen) is associated with the notion of home: nurturing, being

hospitable and supporting others. The earth energy is typically very grounded and stable and the quality of the earth energy is one of rest and revival. If this energy is depleted it manifests itself in behaviour patterns that are often to do with food obsessions, perhaps too much resting or getting stuck in a rut with physical problems to do with digestion, lack of circulation. If in excess, then this may also result in food problems, worrying too much, overworking, with physical symptoms of dryness in the mouth, stomach and ovary problems. This is quite a simplified approach but you can look at the table on page 65 to determine the characteristics of other element imbalances.

Five Element Transformations
The elements interrelate in two different ways. On the one hand they control one another, curbing excess tendencies. So water puts out fire, fire melts metal, metal chops down wood, wood holds together earth, and earth dams up water. This is called the *controlling cycle*. There is also a *creative cycle* in which wood stokes the fire, fire's embers come back to the earth, from within the earth is found metal, metal nourishes water with its minerals, and water is needed by the wood to grow.

If an element is weak you may want to support it or to check it if it is too strong.

Playing with the Elements
In order to embody this somewhat confusing theory you could play a game based on the familiar childhood paper, scissors, stone.
Play this extended version of the game:

Fists (stone) represent earth;
Hand wide (paper) is wood;
Two fingers sideways (scissors) is metal;
Palm up is water;
Four fingers sideways is fire.

You can extend this to a group improvisation where a character moves or reacts to a given situation. Pick elements out of a hat so that no-one knows who the other is playing. Start with pairs initially where you are given a situation of girl-friend/boyfriend argument. Try to work out which element your partner is embodying. Now you may want to extend it to a group situation. It provides the actor with another means of playing with the essence of character much like the traditional archetypes of mother, king, fool and so on.

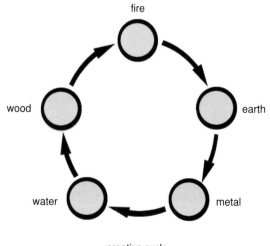

creative cycle

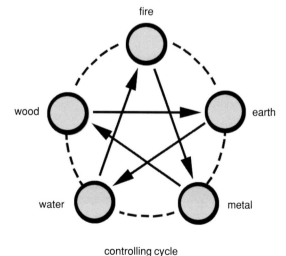

controlling cycle

Controlling and creative cycles in the five elements.

SHIATSU

Shiatsu is Japanese for finger pressure. It is a form of touch therapy that not only uses finger pressure but palms, elbows and knees to stimulate pathways of ki energy in the meridian system. The application of gentle pressure and stretches to the whole body aims to rebalance the meridians, stimulate the body's natural self-healing properties and bring about a re-energized state. On a physical level, Shiatsu is used to help relax the body, relieve aches and pains and promote effective organ function, but it also works to nurture a mind/body connection, which serves to enhance emotional and spiritual wellbeing.

Just as in acupuncture, shiatsu practitioners make use of the pathways of ki energy and the key points along those channels known as 'tsubos' or points. These are small areas accessed by finger or thumb pressure (or needles in acupuncture) that penetrate deeply into the meridian enabling a rebalancing of the energy to take place. Shiatsu embodies an important attitude to medicine, common to many Asian countries, in that it focuses on a preventative approach to illness and attempts to deal with disharmonies in the body before they develop into disease.

Shiatsu is practised fully clothed, normally on the floor on a futon or mat. Sessions last about 60 minutes. Finding the connection with the energy of the client or partner involves the practitioner in harnessing their whole body, mind and most importantly their breath. Crawling techniques are used so that even pressure is applied at a 90 degree angle using gravity and the body's natural weight. Just as in all the other practices we introduce in the book, it is vital to get some hands-on treatment from a qualified practitioner to experience the full power of shiatsu, but there are still a number of ways to benefit from a few partner pressure exercises and some individual work on specific points. In a regular treatment the practitioner would not just work on a single meridian but more holistically, on a combination. However, it is perfectly safe to get a feel for this kind of work particularly when working on the back, which is a fairly robust area. It is also an area that holds a lot of tension that can be diminished with some simple *palming down*.

Avoid working on someone:

- during the early stages of pregnancy;
- if there is a history of serious back problems;
- immediately after eating.

Palming Down the Bladder Meridian

The bladder meridian lies on either side of the spine. Working this area is particularly useful, connecting as it does to our adrenaline that may need firing up or calming down for performance. It also deals with instincts and fears so that tension before performance, in the form of sweats or going to the toilet, can be allayed. Do not do this just before a performance as you will need recovery time. The spine is a vital area as it connects with the nervous system and with the subtle energies of the whole body. Your partner should lie on a futon or mat in prone position (on their stomach) with the head turned to one side. As a preparation, crawl around the space several times, which will give you the sensation of using your body weight in the all-fours position. The crawling action is a very natural, instinctive way of moving that uses a cross-patterning action of the right arm with the left leg and the left arm with the right leg (*see* Chapter 2). As you crawl, bring your attention to the hara by breathing deeply and freeing the neck.

1. Kneel parallel to your partner with your hips in line with theirs, facing towards their head.
2. Take a moment to gather your own energy and breathe deeply into your hara. Bring your hands together and be aware of the energy passing between.
3. Bring your full attention to the person lying next to you and gently place both hands on their sacrum. Take a few moments to connect with their breathing and try to maintain a sympathetic rhythm. On each in breath you should feel a sense of gently releasing and on the out breath you should allow the hands to sink gently into the pull of energy deep within the body. It is important to use your

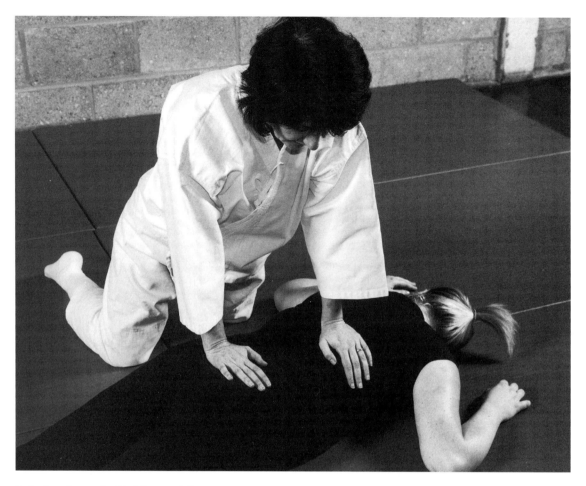

Palming down the bladder meridian.

intention (focusing with the mind/body connection) allowing your hands to feel the magnet force rather than merely applying physical pressure.

4. Now turn your body to face theirs and get into a crawling position with the knees apart, one hand on their sacrum and the other just below the shoulder blade about two finger-widths from the spine on the opposite side.

5. The hand on the sacrum is the Mother hand that stays secure whilst the moving hand is called the Messenger. The very term suggests that it is sending messages to the mother so it is

important to feel this in your intention as you communicate the flow of energy through the hands.

6. Make sure that you are perpendicular to the body and the energy is coming from your hara, not in a forwards direction but as though in a backwards wheel. With this sense of the wheel, lean very gently from your hara into your hands as your partner breathes out, again trying to sense that magnet of energy along the meridian line. As you lean in, bring your body weight over the area you are working on keeping the chest open and the spine long. On

the in breath, release the pressure and move the messenger hand down a few finger-widths toward the mother hand.

7. Continue palming down trying to ensure that your pressure is even between both hands and that you work on the breath. Keep your movement flowing to increase the potential for release. You should also make sure that your hara is always above the area that you are working on, so you will need to move your legs along with the hand movement. Try to remember the crawling action.

8. Once you reach the sacrum repeat the action of palming down the back but this time working on the meridian on the near side, two finger-widths away from the spine, again beginning below the shoulder blades.

9. You can palm in a very slow and measured way if you want to calm the meridian and work a little faster and with more encouraging vitality if you want to stimulate it.

Eight Key Points for Performers

There are a number of very useful points or *tsubo* that may be used by the performer. These are most effective when used as part of a whole treatment but can also be used as self-help particularly in relation to certain conditions. Positions of the points are described using the measuring unit in Traditional Chinese Medicine known as the *cun* or *sun*. This refers to the width of the thumb – but it is always the thumb-width of the body being worked on, not the practitioner's.

Warm up the body with some gentle tapotement all over. Release the wrists so that the hands are floppy and make soft fists to tap or make a percussive action on the fleshy parts of the body to increase circulation and bring the energy to the surface. Alternatively, use the meridian stretches included in the following chapter.

Large Intestine 4
This is a very useful point for all kinds of pain

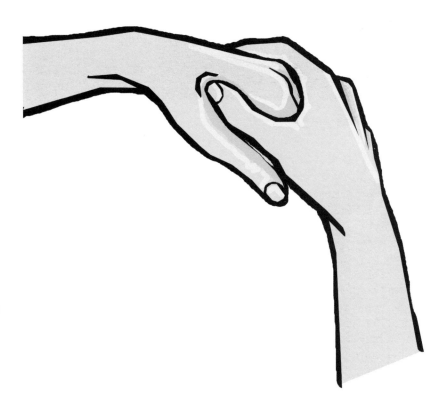

LI 4: In the web between the thumb and index finger, pressing toward the index finger about one cun down on the back of the hand.

69

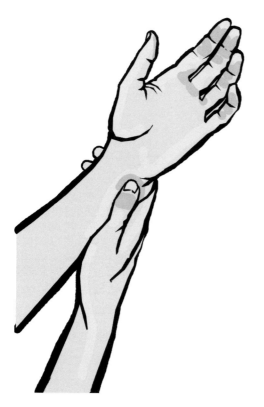

HT 7: On the inside of the wrist just under the bone (palm up, in line with the little finger).

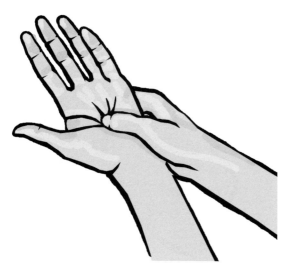

HC 8: In the middle of the palm angled upwards.

relief particularly associated with the head. It is also effective in letting go emotionally and encouraging the body's elimination particularly when feeling bunged up either with constipation or cold.

Heart 7
This meridian has strong associations with the emotions and also with communication. This point is useful for stage fright because it helps to clear the voice and calm the emotions. This point is also good for insomnia.

Heart Constrictor 8
Known as Palace of Anxiety, it is excellent for calming down.

Heart constrictor 6
A well-known point that is used for nausea.

Bladder 2
This helps clear sinus problems and is useful for headaches.

Kidney 1
Known as Gushing Spring, this taps into the energy and is helpful for revitalizing and grounding.

Stomach 36
This is one of the most important points in the body for general wellbeing and is also used for tiredness in the legs.

Liver 3
This is good for detoxing and hangovers.

It can be invaluable for the performer to develop a sensitivity to the nature and fluctuation in their own energy and that of the environment around them. By now, you will have reflected on your own lifestyle and personal tendencies in terms of yin and yang and maybe have a sense of how to balance your energies both for your own personal needs and the requirements of performance. The following chapter offers some opportunities to source the reservoir of energy on a more internal

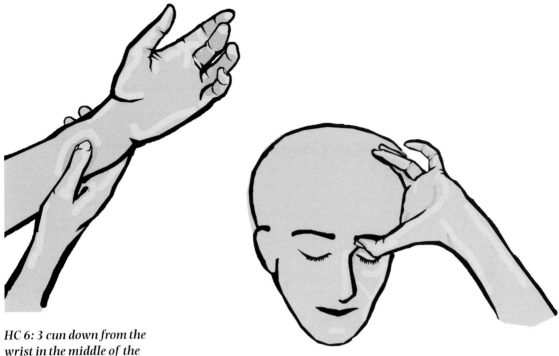

HC 6: 3 cun down from the wrist in the middle of the forearm (palm side).

BL 2: The hollow just inside the inner corner of the eyebrow, angled upward.

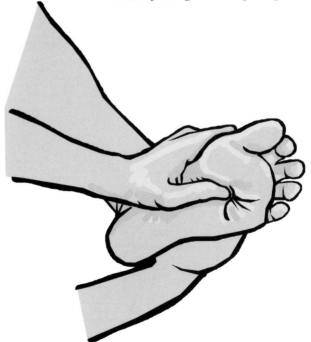

KD 1: Just under the ball of the foot about one-third across under the bulge of the big toe.

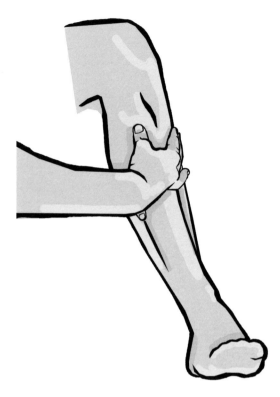

ST 36: About 3 cun under the kneecap, in the muscle on the outer edge of the shin bone.

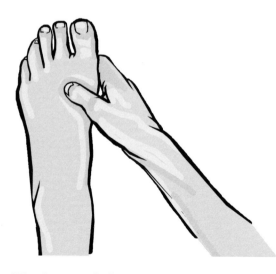

LV 3: Between the big toe and the next about two cun down from the web.

Awareness of the Yin/Yang Exchange

To recap there are several different ways in which an awareness of the yin/yang exchange can be helpful for performers.

• Developing an appreciation of the performer's own yin/yang predisposition and how this may be reshaped in relation to the demands of a role.
• Creating an awareness of the ebb and flow of on-stage interaction that tunes the faculties to 'coming in on the right note'.
• Enabling the choreographer, the conductor or the director to take responsibility for shaping the yin/yang rhythm in the performance as a whole.
• Developing a sensitivity and responsiveness to the yin/yang energies generated by the audience.

---

level. Let us finish yin/yang by assuming the child pose which allows us to restore energy in a very yin manner.

Child Pose
This is a yoga pose that is often used as a recovery position in between bouts of very yang activity. It is so called because children often rest in this position.

1. Kneel with your bottom on your thighs or with a cushion between your thighs and calves.
2. Breathe in lengthening the spine and on the exhalation, incline forward over your thighs, bending at the hips keeping long on the front of the body.
3. If you feel comfortable, rest your forehead on the ground.
4. Arms can either be resting on the floor alongside the body or stretched out above the head on the floor.
5. As an alternative leg position, you can open the knees and lower the body onto the ground between, giving a welcome opening to the shoulders.

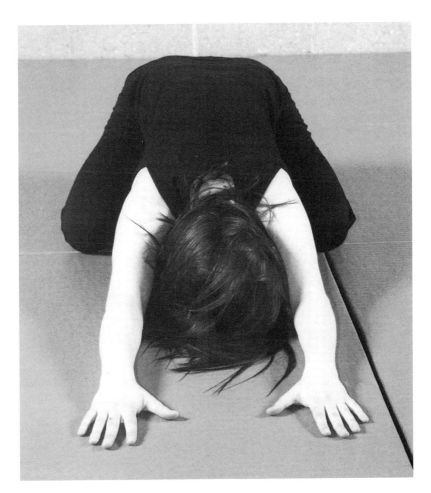

Resting in child pose.

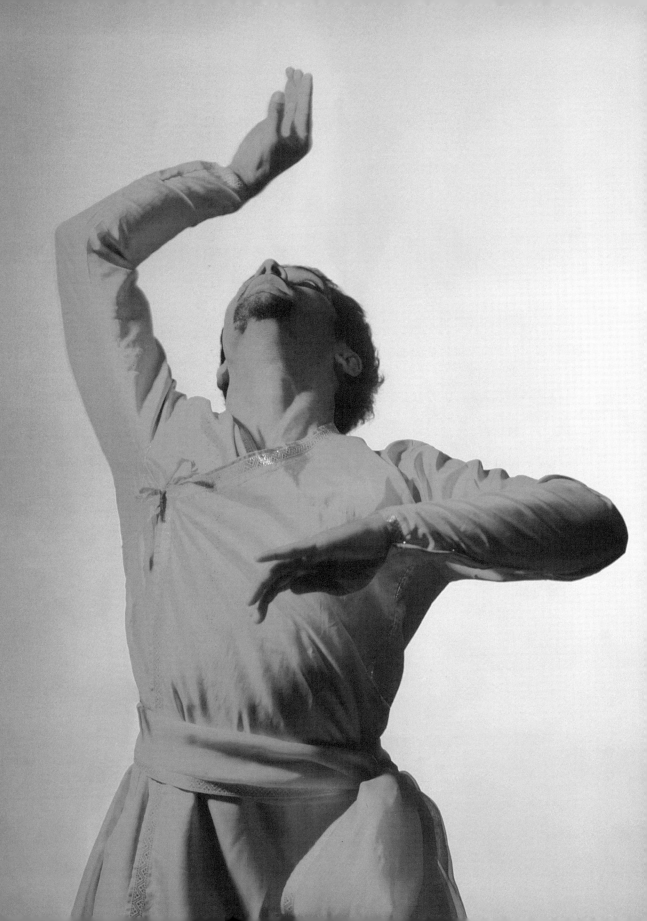

4 DIVINING ENERGY SOURCES

The word *divining* is a reference to the practice of finding water, armed only with a highly developed sensitivity and a hazel twig. By using different bodywork practices, we can learn to feel, kinaesthetically and on the breath, the pull of the energy and bring it to the surface, like the diviner. The practice of yoga has for centuries been a vital source of energy whose potential has only recently begun to be tapped by westerners. Many training schools and theatre companies now harness yoga as a means of developing the skills of their performers and to enhance the mind/body dialogue. As well as considering yoga's regenerating powers, we also explore two related methods of sourcing energy, the *meridians* and the *chakras*. These are characterized by special visualizations or maps, that, in conjunction with breathing, movement and sounding, allow us to draw energy from ancient tributaries deep within the body. In the process, blocked energy is released and the entire being is replenished.

As a preliminary to sourcing energy in the body through yoga, let us just feel our own energy at the surface.

Feel the Force
Rub your hands together vigorously until you feel heat and sensation rising to the surface. Now separate your palms by just a centimetre or two and without touching the hands together, bounce them back and forth feeling the force of the energy you have just generated. Keep thinking of the tension of an elastic band and tease your hands further and further away until you have a ball of

OPPOSITE: *Akram Khan – Magnetic energy in performance.* Photographer *Chris Nash*

energy between them. If you go too quickly you will lose the magnetic pull, so return to rubbing your hands vigorously.

Having felt the power between your own palms, you can extend this exercise to partner work by placing your palms almost touching. Once you have felt the energy between you, try taking the palms further apart and see if you can still feel the connection. Energy emanates not just at the surface of the skin but radiates beyond. It is this quality of expansion that is so vital to the performer's ability to communicate: it is the star's ability to shine.

YOGA

The principles of classical yoga were laid out by the Indian scholar Patanjali in his text *The Eight Limbs of Yoga* some 2,000 years ago. Yoga means 'union' referring to the union of body, mind and spirit. Authentic yoga systems must involve *all three* aspects – anything less is an imitation. In all the major schools there is an emphasis on the value of *mindful breathing*, as a vital means of making the connection between body, mind and spirit. In classical yoga the physical postures are called *asanas* and these are practised to prepare the body for *pranayama*, the name given to the meditative breathing practice. In the West, yoga has been widely practised by performers since Stanislavski and has become increasingly influential over the last fifty years.

There are a bewildering number of styles and systems of yoga now on offer and as many dedicated and skilful teachers. Some methods have quite specific approaches to the sourcing of energy. It is probably best to try out several methods before committing to one system. You may discover features from a variety of approaches that you will use according to your different needs. As with all body work, it is desirable to find a suitable class as this will help you to deepen your own practice. It is worth remembering that yoga is essentially the union of *body, mind and spirit* and although the mere outward execution of a posture may bring some sense of physical achievement, it will not allow you to become fully sensitized to the body's energy sources. Only through harnessing the breath and maintaining a physical mindfulness of the relationship of the dan tien to the rest of the body, can the practice develop to its full potential. Given below are some of the defining features of several significant contemporary schools of yoga.

The Iyengar Method

The Iyengar method was one of the first methods to be practised on a large scale in the West. There is still a great respect for the system of teaching developed by B.K.S. Iyengar, with its reputation for thoroughness and a meticulous understanding of the body. It takes discipline to practise in the classic Iyengar way – *asanas* have to be held for a considerable length of time and there is an emphasis on strictly extended limbs. This is demanding for the beginner whose muscles may initially protest. It's important to be able to distinguish pain from strong sensation and to learn to ease off when your body tells you it has had enough. One of the great benefits of this system is that in maintaining a posture for some time, working through some of the initial barriers of tension and restlessness can

take you to a place where, through breathing, you begin to connect at a very deep level with what is occurring in the mind and body. This discipline of holding the pose enables one to be present in the moment, in a very Alexander way. At this level, you are sourcing the energy.

A particular benefit of the Iyengar system is the recommended use of props that can help the untutored body get the feeling of an *asana*, even if the body is a long way from being able to achieve the full potential of the pose. Belts, blocks and chairs are variously used to support the body and give a sense of the direction in which the body should be moving. Beginners often get demoralized when the body seems to be stuck in a position; the following gives a sample of just a few of the more challenging *asanas* that can be developed by using supportive props according to the Iyengar method. These give the body a chance to stay in the position without strain.

Standing Forward Bend, Resting on Chair-Back
This is a good preparation for forward bending and excellent for feeling what is happening in the back during the early days of forward bending positions. It is much less of an extreme stretch on the hamstrings than the conventional sitting forward bend, so allows for the spine to begin to lengthen without too much interference from agonized legs. If the spine is allowed to lengthen, then the energy can flow freely.

1. Stand hip-width apart at about a metre's distance from the back of a chair.
2. Breathe in and as you exhale stretch the arms forwards placing the palms of the hands on the chair back.
3. Stretch away with the hands and back with the hips to encourage length in the trunk. Check that you are positioned the right distance from the chair. Your legs should be vertical with the hips over the ankles.
4. Sense if there are any raised vertebrae on the spine and gently take the attention and breath into this area to ease out stiffness. You can try bending and then stretching the legs to encourage more sensation and length in

Releasing the spine in standing forward bend.

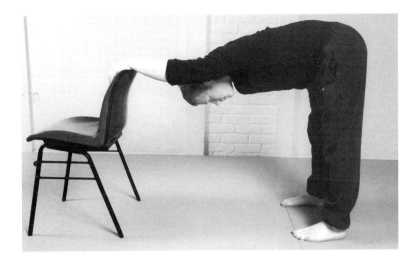

these trouble spots, releasing forward on the exhalation.

5. If, on the other hand, you feel any areas of the back sinking, allow this area to rise up slightly, bringing the vertebrae in line, creating a long, level back.

6. Keep breathing your way into the pose. You can even ask a partner to observe the lie of your spine and to gently place their fingers on any areas of tension. Breathe into their fingers to see if you can bring about a release.

Supported Sitting Forward Bend

The sitting forward bend is another potentially rewarding asana that many people give up on because it can feel very uncomfortable until the body has learned to release forward. The following Iyengar technique provides a way of progressing and benefiting from the asana, in relative comfort. The common obstacle to improvement in the forward bend is because the pelvis doesn't tilt forward sufficiently and people can't feel the bend from the very base of the spine. This supported method helps the pelvis to find the initial forward bending direction.

1. Sit on a rolled up blanket or wedge.

2. Inhale and as you exhale begin to incline the trunk forward, sensing the movement coming from low down at the base of the spine, rather than in the mid-back.

3. Resist the temptation to nose-dive and try and keep the length on the spine. With each inhalation ease off the stretch in the legs. With each exhalation release the body weight forwards and feel the heels lengthening away. Focus on the navel area as you exhale and think of it moving back and up towards the pelvis.

4. Reach out, and maintaining your length, support the arms on a chair or low stool. With your elbows light and slightly lifted, try and maintain the thought that the spine is in a long line and rest forward in this position.

5. Try activating the legs by flexing the feet on the exhalation. This may help you to slide forward on your thighs.

6. Another useful thought is to soften the neck as you forward bend. Too often we try and hoist ourselves forward by sheer willpower and when we do so the neck tightens and the whole body contracts. The aim is to avoid any contraction so that the energy flows freely.

Inverted Poses

Now we move into some inverted poses that take the body from its customary upright position to upside down. This has enormous health benefits as energy is shaken up and the arteries of the body are relieved of their usual uphill struggle to return blood to the heart. This can create a surge of energy that can be profoundly restorative. For the beginner, these inverted poses can be a little

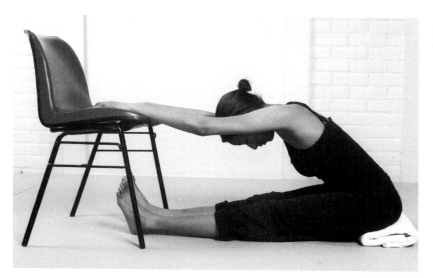

Supported sitting forward bend.

disturbing for the body but start slowly and build up. These poses should not be practised during menstruation or pregnancy.

Shoulder Stand, Queen of Asanas
This asana can be notoriously uncomfortable until the upper spine and shoulders have developed the strength and flexibility to support a relatively upright upside-down position. Until then, and whilst the back is bowed and the legs struggle to find the vertical, the neck is likely to be constricted, causing shortening of the breath and pressure in the eyes. All this can be avoided with the recommended Iyengar use of a chair and a blanket to support the body whilst it develops mobility and balance. Choose a strong chair with sturdy frame.

1. Fold a blanket several times being careful to smooth out any creases in the fabric. Arrange yourself on the blanket so that your head is at ground level with the neck supported by the folds of the blanket when upside down. Lie symmetrically, lengthening your neck before placing your head down.
2. Roll your hips off the ground and raise your legs up and over your head, arriving with your toes towards the floor behind you.
3. Get a friend to place a chair with its seat facing you a short distance behind your back.

4. Reach your forearms through the chair legs to grip the back legs.
5. Now roll your trunk and legs back over towards the chair and place your sacrum on the front edge of the chair.
6. From this position, you can either extend your legs vertically into the air or alternatively bring your calves carefully down to rest on the back of the chair and rest in this supported position. Either way, your forearms, arms, and torso will be supported by the chair-legs and frame.
7. If you press the arms down into the ground, you will find that the body is able to lift up far more easily away from this point of gravity.
8. From this position you can work to lift the chest, gaining the benefits of shoulder stand that both draws from and sends energy to the circulatory, endocrine, digestive and respiratory systems.

Practising in this way, you will be able to hold the asana much longer than in a collapsed, free-standing position. In time, you can dispense with the chair if this feels right for you. However, the blanket (or foam block if you are using one) will protect your neck and make you feel much more comfortable, even when you are able to do the asana without other support.

The Plough

This is often done after holding the shoulder stand for a while and activating the upper back in that preliminary position. It is a useful way of strengthening the back prior to attempting a headstand. As the legs are taken over the head, energy flows freely to the brain, clearing the mind. Again, there is an Iyengar method of supporting the pose. Before beginning the asana, arrange the blanket and chair as in the photograph.

1. Place the head and neck carefully on the floor with the shoulders on the rolled blanket, as for the shoulder stand, above.
2. Lift the hips and spine and, keeping elbows tucked in, use the blades of your hands to support the upper spine.
3. Swing legs over in a controlled way to arrive on the chair, as shown in the photograph below.
4. From this position, and pressing the hands into the back to get more purchase and height on the back, it is possible to lift the spine so that you become as vertical as possible between the hips and shoulder. Lift the sitting bones up and again, press the upper arms into the ground, to create more lift on the spine.
5. In the early stages of practising the plough, the chair will ensure that you do not exert too extreme a stretch on the back, which might cause the back to bow outwards. In time you

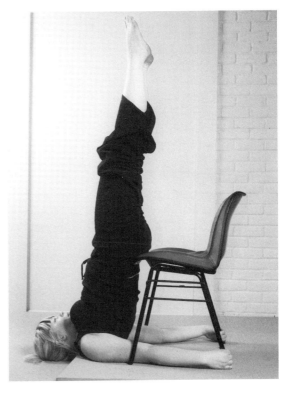

Supported shoulder stand.

will be able to use lower levels of chair until you have achieved the full plough position with feet touching the ground.

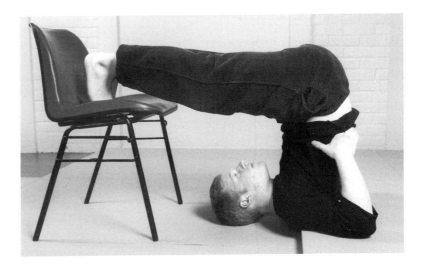

Supported plough.

Ashtanga Yoga

Ashtanga Yoga is a reference to and translation of Patanjali's 'Eight Limbs of Yoga'. The system, originally developed by Patthabhi Jois is now taught by a rapidly growing number of western teachers. In recent years, the Ashtanga method has proved particularly influential, gaining many advocates, especially amongst the young, fit and energetic. It is a highly *dynamic* yoga system consisting of flowing poses in which the asanas are performed in a strict sequence, according to a carefully regulated breathing pattern. It is a challenging system but one relished by devotees, partly for its yang-like characteristics of activity and fiery heat that are said to burn off many of the body toxins and impurities, creating in the participant a feeling of purification and strong energy. Ashtanga yoga works on the cardio-vascular system since the *asanas* are linked by strenuous jumps working the heart, lungs and entire muscular-skeletal structure of the body. Many people report a dramatically improved sense of wellbeing after practising; undoubtedly this is partly due to the endomorphs released and the general strengthening of the body systems. It is a good method for those who are already quite fit and flexible and those working with energetic performance demands.

The Ashtanga practice is organized around three graded series or levels of difficulty. The movements are learned in a strict order with the breath, and flow from one to the other on the inhalation and exhalation. The idea is that asanas ride on the breath without strain. For many, working in this ordered way provides a familiar structure through which to monitor progress and develop flexibility, stamina and endurance. Having mastered the basic sequences of asanas and breath, the student is encouraged to develop their own *Self-Practice*. Many classes at this level take the form of the student's own self-directed process through the Series whilst the teacher offers guidance and makes adjustments to the asanas. This can provide a very valuable way of developing one's practice.

As you advance in Ashtanga practice, you will be introduced to a way of channelling energy through a combination of breathing and an awareness of the bandhas. The three *bandhas* are described as key *energetic locks*, found in the throat, the lower abdomen and at the root of the torso (between the anus and the perineum). Learning to engage with and draw up the bandhas whilst executing the asanas, takes committed practice under the tuition of an Ashtanga teacher. As in all serious yoga systems, there is a strong emphasis in Ashtanga yoga on the crucial role played by the dan tien area (approximating to the central bandha), in supporting the practice.

Sun Salutation

In the Ashtanga system, this is an important vinyasa that is always performed several times at the beginning of yoga practice and is used extensively to link together various sequences of asanas. *Sun Salutation* takes the body through a range of releasing and strengthening movements and can be intensely energizing. Because it is so physically demanding, there is a real sense of the lungs and heart being deeply engaged in the work. There are two versions of Sun Salutation performed in Ashtanga yoga. The version given here is known as Sun Salutation A. It is important that the movements flow from one to another without interruption and following the specified breathing. It's a sequence that takes years to perfect but provides a fundamental preparation for much of the more advanced work on the body. Performed regularly, it creates a discipline in the body and mind that is enormously strengthening. Some of the asanas involved in Sun Salutation, are explored in more detail later in the chapter under the heading, *A Soft Approach*. You may wish to revisit this vinyasa when you have deepened your understanding of the basic movements.

1. Assume the standing pose with feet in parallel.
2. Inhale as you stretch the arms above the head and look up towards the sky.
3. On the exhalation fold into a standing forward bend, keeping the legs long but not hitting back on the knees.

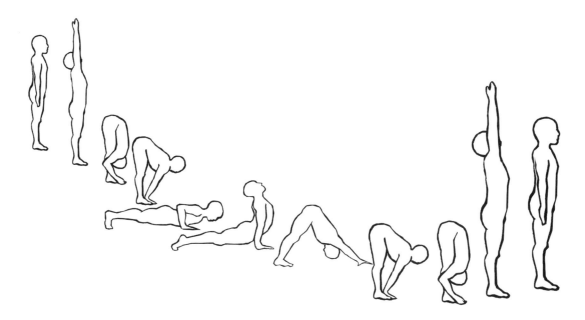

Ashtanga sun salutation A.

4. Keeping the fingertips touching the ground, inhale as you extend the head up, leading from the brow centre. Keep the spine long and the neck free.
5. Exhale as you place the palms on the floor to either side of your feet (you may need to bend your knees) and jump the feet back, tucking the elbows in. Keep the body as long and straight as you can in what is called plank position with the hands and the feet supporting the body. Try not to let the bottom sag down but focus on trying to keep the body in a straight line from heels to head.
6. Inhale and move the body forward by rolling over the toes and looking up, lifting the head and breastbone. This action will allow the upper spine to lift up away from the floor. Support by pressing the hands down strongly into the ground, allowing the shoulders to relax and drop down.
7. From this position, exhale as you push backwards into downward dog with your bottom lifting up towards the ceiling. Your weight is now supported between your hands and your feet and. Take three deep breaths, drawing the navel towards the waist on the exhalation. Allow yourself to sink simultaneously into your legs and your hands, allowing the spine to lengthen and release between these points of extension.
8. On an in breath jump the feet back to point 4, repeating the action of the head looking upwards with fingertips touching the ground.
9. Exhale into the standing forward bend described in point 3.
10. As you inhale, unfold the trunk so that you return to standing with arms lifted above the head (point 2).
11. Resume the standing position (point 1), ready to begin again.
12. You should aim to perform the sun salutation five times.

A 'Soft' Contemporary Approach to the Classic Asanas

In recent years, there has been a shift in the thinking of some classically trained teachers towards developing what might be called *a softer approach* to the practice of yoga, one more in line with the principles of the *soft body* (*see* Hard and Soft Stretch, and the Alexander Technique in Chapters 1 and 2). According to this 'new' style, pioneered by Vanda Scaravelli, amongst other important contributors, students are especially encouraged to *feel* what is going on in their bodies from moment to moment and discover for themselves, how to make space and length in the body through a process of kinaesthetic experimentation. This may involve holding back from going into a completed version of the asana until the body is ready and has found the appropriate length and space. Within some classes of this 'new' approach to yoga, the student may be encouraged to decide when to enter and exit from asanas, and to work the body in alternating pairs of asanas (see below), moving from one to the other to engage the body in a gentle counter-stretching process and really tuning in to the sensations of working the body.

Conventional approaches to yoga encourage the participant to stretch the body to its full extent by going immediately into the asana as deeply as possible. According to the less orthodox approach, the limbs are not held rigidly in straight lines, bracing the poses, but are sometimes held more softly while the pose is being explored, even though the base of the poses may be anchored securely into the ground. The emphasis is not in achieving the completed asana, but in journeying, working sympathetically with the body to encourage the free flow of energy and never using the limbs to forcibly hoist the pose into position. The crucial aim is to avoid tensing and forcing the body into a fixed end position that only serves to block energy.

Although in this method, there may be an increased feeling of ownership of the body through the freedom to experiment, this in no way implies a loss of discipline. In fact, the onus to test out the principles of the practice in and on the body, brings with it a great sense of responsibility, rather than simply 'copying' a master. We are indebted to Bill Wood and his teachers for an introduction to this progressive approach.

The Wave

The focus of this work is on allowing the lower spine to release downwards, so that the upper body can lift upwards. This is partly achieved by encouraging the navel to move in towards the spine on the exhalation which has the effect of softening and lengthening the lumbar spine in the waist area. This extension of the lower spine releases the vertebrae in other, generally stiffer parts of the upper spine. Scaravelli described this action as having the quality of a 'wave'. This sense of the wave begins with an awareness of gravity and our body's strong contact with the ground, which allows us to release upwards and away. In every asana the attention is on the central core of the body. There is still a real attention on the body *rooting* itself into the ground through the contact of the feet (or back foot), so that the spine and upper body are free to lengthen away from this point of resistance. The best way to feel the effects of this approach in and on one's own body, is to try out these principles in some key asanas as follows.

Fierce Pose

The power of this asana is often underestimated. Practised in a mindful way, the *fierce pose* can be immensely effective in releasing the lumbar spine. In time, this action improves the entire alignment and wellbeing of the body. It brings about a subtle adjustment of the spine in relation to the pelvis opening up more space and making available an improved blood supply to the abdominal organs and releasing energy throughout the area. Although the name of the pose suggests a very yang quality, this can be achieved more effectively with the 'soft' approach.

1. Stand with feet hip-width apart, toes a little in from the heels and place the hands in prayer position.
2. Breathe in and as you breathe out, bend the knees a little.
3. Resist the impulse to collapse in the waist and instead focus on dropping your sacrum downwards as if it were a lead weight at the bottom of a plumb line.

RIGHT: *Fierce pose with lumbar spine collapsed.*

FAR RIGHT: *Softer method of fierce pose.*

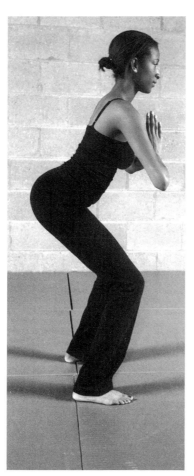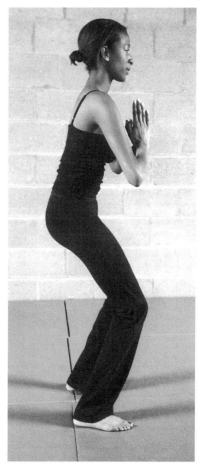

4. On the exhalation, allow your navel to move back and in towards the spine. This will help to release the lower back.
5. Keep adjusting the position, alternating between standing and bending the knees, as you lengthen and soften the waist. Resist the impulse to tip too far forwards in the trunk.

Fierce pose is often carried out in conjunction with the standing forward bend that follows. When you feel tired in one asana, alternate to the other paired asana to allow recovery time and to benefit from the counter-stretch.

'Soft' Standing Forward Bend
The unique aspect about the asana taught in the 'soft' way is that the legs do not have to be braced into a rigid position. The knees may be gently bent to allow the spine to lengthen though the sensation should still be of the soles of the feet firmly making contact with the ground.

1. Stand with feet in parallel slightly apart. Breathe in.
2. As you exhale, fold the trunk forwards towards the floor from the hips softening the knees as necessary. Do not nose-dive but think instead of keeping the length in your spine.
3. Keeping the head in line with the spine and allowing room behind the knees, let the waist lengthen and soften each time you exhale, drawing the navel in and up, like a bubble rising in a bottle. Think of your body weight engaging through your shoulders and into

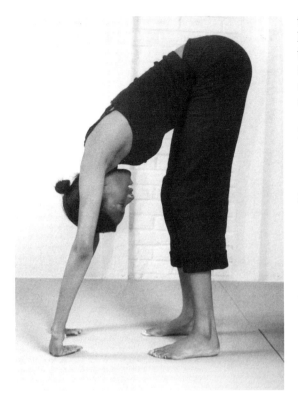

Soft standing forward bend.

your extended arms as you rest the fingers into the floor.

4. Maintaining this length on the spine, allow the feeling of a continuous line from the sacrum to the crown of the head and through into the arms. Keep the neck soft. Remember not to tighten the shoulder blades as you rest down into the fingertips on the floor. The shoulders should feel as though they are moving down and away from the head.

Downward Dog

This asana is one of the cornerstones of the yoga practice as we saw in the Sun Salutation A (common to both Iyengar and Ashtanga methods). As described here, it is a pose in which one can stay for a while, before moving in and out of the two 'soft' versions of the poses detailed above. *Downward Dog* is practised effectively by sensing the relationship between the spine and the limbs, so

that in this approach the knees may be soft and not locked. Feet press firmly into the ground, even if the heels are not resting on the floor. You can alternate this position to good effect with *fierce pose* and *soft standing forward bend*. Use a yoga mat to avoid slipping.

1. First organize yourself in the downward dog position with feet hip-width apart, buttock bones to the sky and the hands shoulder-width apart, pressing feet strongly into the ground.
2. As with the standing forward bend, the legs should be long but not at the expense of tightening up the back. If the hamstrings are tight, try releasing the knees slightly and, instead, see if you can feel a lengthening in the spine.
3. Don't let yourself get stuck in *Dog Pose* or you may find yourself hanging mindlessly on the stretch. Allow yourself some exploratory movement both of the breath and the body. For example, try making some little circles with the pelvis to free up the position or experiment with Scaravelli's recommendation to 'gallop like a horse' on the spot, an action that really gives a sense of the quadruped movement and helps to engage the shoulders.
4. It's really important to give your weight to the floor through the hands and feet. The hands should feel alive. Keep experimenting to find the sensation of lengthening in the spine. This is your energy source.
5. Some yoga methods advocate sinking the shoulders to the point where the head is resting on the floor. Instead, keep the spine in line with the shoulders and focus instead on lengthening the waist, working with the breath to soften and draw this area in on the exhalation. The more you are able to find this action, the more the stiffness in the vertebrae will begin to unravel. You have the feeling that you are hanging from the belly button that floats up towards the spine on each exhalation. The chest and rib cage feel as though they are hanging from the spine.
6. Listen to your body and as soon as you feel you have done enough, move into one of the other

poses in this section, and keep shifting between the three, each time discovering a deeper energetic quality.

This 'new' approach can have a profound effect on the individual and though apparently 'easier', it encourages a deep release and contact with energy sources. An effective flow of energy can be nurtured by working with sensations to release the body and avoiding the tensions of *end-gaining* in a locked pose. From these fundamental poses, the performer's body becomes sensitized, as the effort of movement is distilled and physical articulation becomes more fluent.

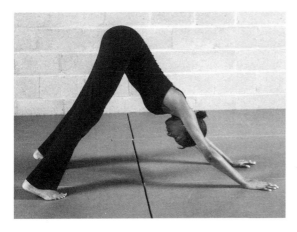

Downward dog.

Masunaga Makka-ho Stretches

The previous chapter introduced the mapping of the body into meridian lines through the practice of shiatsu. Apart from receiving treatments from a trained practitioner there are other ways to encourage the performer to boost and balance their own distribution of ki energy through these pathways. The Japanese shiatsu master, Masunaga, developed a series of self-help stretches to nurture the flow of energy that in turn improve breathing and organ function and rebalance the body. These stretches are performed by working the meridians in their elemental pairs identified in the Five Element chart in Chapter 3. When working the stretches it is more important that you do not force

the body but use the stretch to gain an awareness of what is happening within. It is vital to visualize the route of meridians as you perform the stretch so that you start to sensitize your body to the energy channel being released. The stretches are very demanding so it's important not to push beyond your physical limits. The idea is not to prove how flexible you are but to gauge how contracted or depleted the energy flow may be in your own body.

Through regular practice, the performer will really start to feel which stretches they find most difficult at different moments in their life. Tighter meridians will often be blocked or overactive. The practice can become a tool of self-diagnosis as the performer learns to identify that perhaps if the stretch is easier than normal then the meridians may be a little lacking in energy flow and need some stimulus by holding the stretch for longer. It is important to breathe deeply into the stretches and release on the outbreath. Hold each position for three or four deep breaths. They should be done in the order listed as they mirror the flow of energy through the day. It is important to perform the entire sequence in order to balance all the meridians.

Lung/Large Intestine = Metal
1. Place your hands behind you, link thumbs, and point your index fingers downward. Legs are slightly wider than hip-width with feet slightly angled inwards.
2. Now lengthen your spine and on the out breath lower the torso from the hips so that the head moves toward the feet and the arms reach upward. Try to feel a widening across the chest as the arms pull backward and feel the extension running along the back of the legs. Hold and breathe.
3. Slowly raise the body from the hips keeping the length of the spine and allow the arms to lower.
4. You should repeat the stretch linking the thumbs the opposite way to even out the chest expansion. When you release from this stretch you may feel a tingling along the meridian as the energy is activated. You may even feel the arms wanting to float upwards a little.

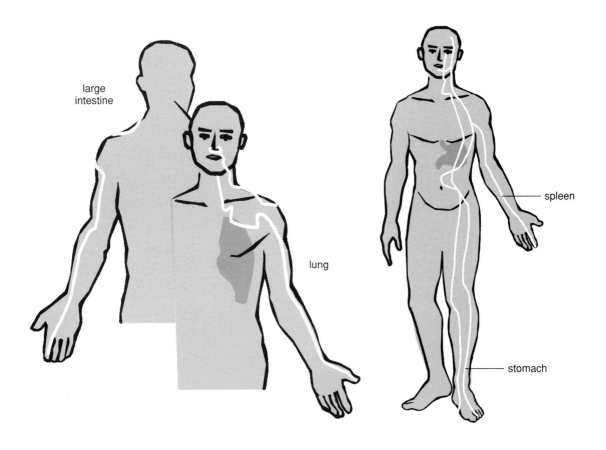

large
intestine

lung

spleen

stomach

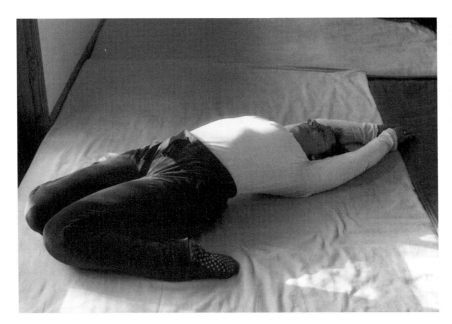

ABOVE LEFT:
**Lung/large intestine
meridian.**

ABOVE RIGHT:
**Stomach/spleen
meridians.**

**Stomach/spleen
stretch.**

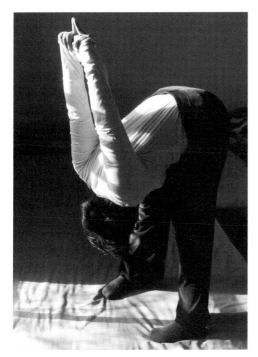

Lung/large intestine stretch.

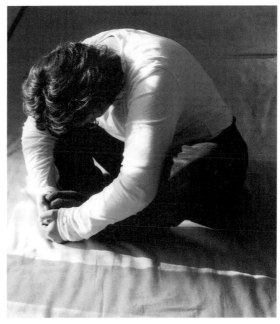

Heart/small intestine stretch.

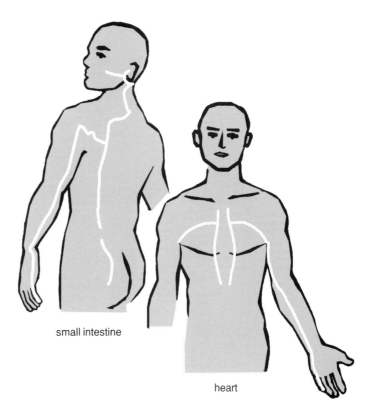

small intestine

heart

Heart/small intestine meridians.

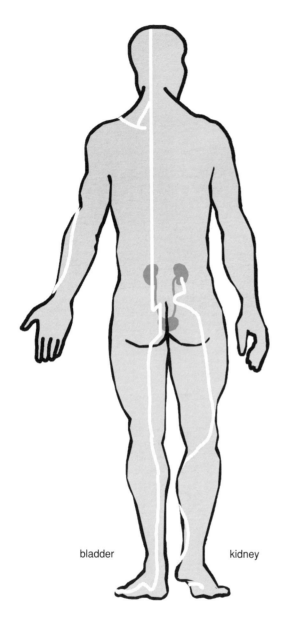

Bladder/kidney meridians.

Stomach/Spleen = Earth

1. Kneel with your feet slightly outside your bottom. Lower your body slowly backwards by leaning onto your elbows. This may be a sufficient stretch for most people. Hold and breathe.

2. Only if you are ready and without pain in the knees, slowly lower your body until your shoulders, head and back come to rest on the floor. Eventually your arms can come to rest above the head.

3. Breathe into the pose, visualizing the meridian lines particularly along the front of the thighs and upwards though the chest to the jaw and temples.

4. This is a very challenging pose so do not hesitate to use supports. You can put a cushion under your knees and one between your calves and thighs. Just by leaning back onto your hands placed by your feet you may experience enough of a stretch in this area.

Heart/ Small Intestine = Fire

1. Sit on the floor with the soles of your feet together and knees open. Try to sit with your spine as straight as you can, so think about your hips sinking into the floor. You can sit on a block or several blankets to encourage the knees to fall.

2. Your elbows need to be opened out as you hold the soles of your feet with your little fingers by your big toe and your thumbs around the front of the foot.

3. Keeping the spine in line, allow the body to incline forwards letting the head extend forward, lengthening the stretch by allowing the elbows to open forward and outward. Release your body weight towards the ground so that your knees open further. Hold and breathe.

4. Think of the meridian lines running from under your armpits down to your little finger and along the inside of your leg to underneath your heel as you stretch and breathe.

Bladder/ Kidney = Water

This is the yoga sitting forward bend that we explored earlier in the chapter that can be performed with the help of a blanket and chair if required.

1. Sitting on the floor, extend your legs straight in front of you. Take your arms to above your head and stretch the spine upwards.

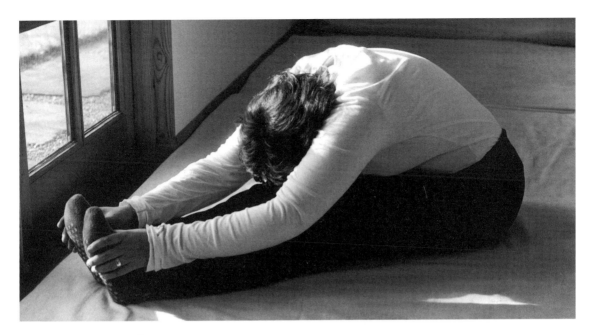

Bladder/kidney stretch.

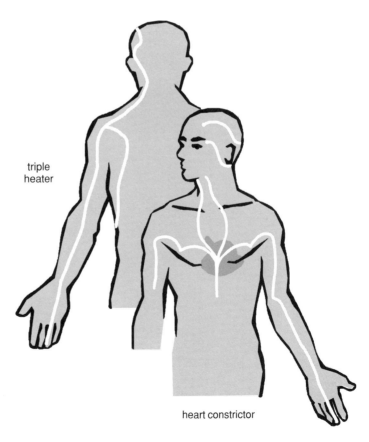

triple
heater

heart constrictor

*Triple heater/heart constrictor
meridians.*

89

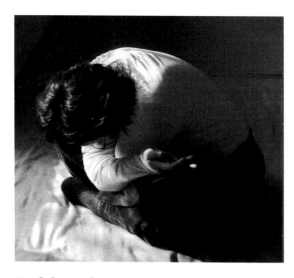

Triple heater/heart constrictor stretch.

2. Incline forward from the hips with the spine without collapsing the spine and lengthen your arms forward toward your feet. Don't allow your chin to push toward the feet or the hands to grab them. Hold and breathe.
3. The stretch is in visualizing the meridians running from your head starting from the eyebrow, down either side of the spine and along the backs of your legs.

Triple Heater/Heart Meridian = Supplemental Fire
1. In sitting position, cross your legs (right over left) and cross your arms (right over left) and lean forward and downwards.
2. Visualize a stretch from the shoulder blades down the outside of the arms to the tips of the fingers, and on the outside of the legs. This is a position that can be repeated crossing left over right with arms and legs.

Liver/Gall Bladder = Wood
1. Sit with legs extended outwards.
2. Raise your arms above your head to lengthen the spine and rotate the torso slightly to the right. This will give you the space to lean back over to the left side of the body.
3. Feel the stretch all down the right side of the arms and torso. You will also feel it in your legs on the inside from the groin down and on the outside. Hold and breathe and repeat on the other side of the body.
4. You must make sure that you keep the torso straight, keep the shoulders back and do not allow the body to collapse in order to reach further to the side. It is better to extend the body only 10 degrees to one side and feel the stretch in the side of the body rather than using the head or arms to reach out towards the feet (*see* the photograph opposite).

Chakras

Common to Hindu, Buddhist and Taoism philosophies, and frequently associated with yoga, the *chakras* are wheels of energy located along the length of the body. The principal seven are found between the base of the spine and just above the

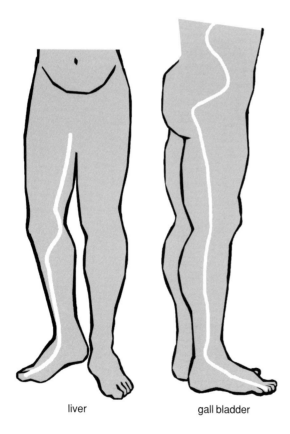

liver   gall bladder

Liver/gall bladder meridians.

Liver/gall bladder stretch.

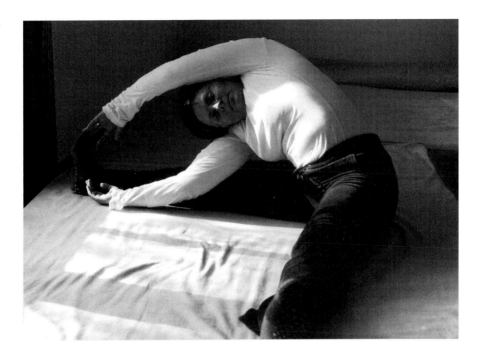

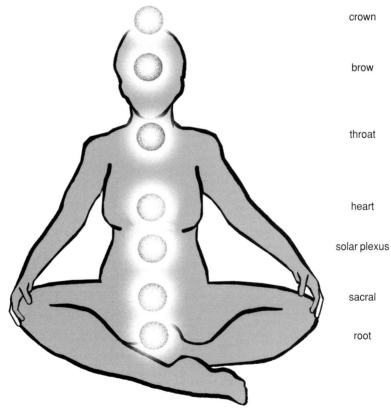

crown

brow

throat

heart

solar plexus

sacral

root

The chakras.

head. These chakras are said to be the bridge between the spiritual and physical worlds. They move energy by spinning and so transform universal energy (prana) into spiritual energy. Freeing the chakras confers specific psychological and physical benefits and opens the channels of creativity much like the meridian system of Traditional Chinese Medicine. The chakras build on one another so that imbalances in the lower chakras can affect the health of those that rest upon them. The illustration on page 91 shows the chakras as they occur along the spine that significantly houses the central nervous system affecting the entire body. Each chakra is associated with specific colours that act as outward symbols helping us to connect with the internal. These are the colours of the rainbow.

The following sequence takes you through each of the seven chakras by means of yoga asanas and breathing techniques linked in with vocal sounds to activate the chakra energy. The power of the chanting voice is seen to stimulate the energy of the chakra that then vibrates and transforms negative emotions. It is important to remember that yoga is intrinsically linked to a religious system so that the energy of the chakra can be raised by wholesome thought transmitted through meditation. The release of such positive energy has the effect of uncoiling the chakra wheel, whereas the presence of negative energy can lock the wheel shut. An understanding of the psycho-physical properties of each of the chakras can help you identify where your own energy blocks may exist. As the sound waves are released during the vocalization, the clarity of the resonance gives us an indication of the state of the chakra.

Some preparation notes:

- The sequence should be followed starting with the root chakra.
- Each stage takes you through an asana, followed by a colour visualization and the release of a sound or mantra.
- Some of the asanas are explored earlier in the chapter where more detailed guidelines are given.
- For the visualization and mantra you will return to a comfortable sitting position (ideally cross-legged and ultimately lotus). It is essential to maintain a long spine so use firm cushions if necessary.
- For each mantra it is important to release the sound on an extended breath, holding the note steady for as long as is comfortable. Repeat this several times, sensing the vibration in the region of the chakra.
- If you have difficulty visualizing colours it is helpful to think of an object or precious stone of that colour.

Base or Root Chakra

This is located at the base of the spine or the perineum and is red. Its energy is connected with primal instincts to do with animal survival and grounding. Associated physical properties are the large intestine, legs, kidneys and adrenals (the adrenaline rush of flight or fight). An underactive base chakra energy would result in feeling timid and ungrounded. An excess of energy would result in rather aggressive behaviour. The following asana is a variation of the forward bend.

1. To access the base chakra, sit with the left leg outstretched and the right foot tucked into the groin.
2. Extend the spine upwards and over the outstretched leg. This helps to activate the whole spine and particularly the coccyx.
3. Return to a cross-legged position on the floor and really feel yourself sinking into your sitting bones so that you are strongly rooted.
4. You may try walking on your sitting bones to intensify the feeling of groundedness.
5. Bringing your attention to the base of the spine, focus on the colour red. Inhale and on the exhalation make the sound 'o' as in pole.

You may find sounding the mantras a little strange, but think of it as an internal massage stimulating the area with vibration created through sound. Tapping into pre-linguistic sounds helps us get in touch with our instincts and the unique properties of each chakra. How strongly does the sound resonate? Do you have difficulty getting any power into this area or does it feel very natural? Be bold in your vocalizations, you will get much better feedback from your body.

Sacral Chakra

This is located in the sacrum. Orange in colour, it is identified with nourishment and sexual pleasure. Anyone with any eating problems may suffer imbalances in this area. The corresponding body parts are the reproductive system and the bladder/kidney function. The healthy sacral chakra nurtures warm generosity in a person. Neglect can result in moods and depression.

1. Assume the cat pose (Chapter 2).
2. Bring your attention to the sacrum as you undulate the spine.
3. Return to sitting crossed-legged visualizing orange. Inhale and on an exhalation sound an 'oo' as in root.

Solar Plexus Chakra

This is located beneath the ribcage in the centre of the chest. This is a very strong area that is traditionally associated with being the emotional centre. The colour is yellow and the energy is associated with confidence, success and achievement. The physical correspondence is the digestive system and liver/gallbladder. This is the area that would be affected in people who tend to act the victim, or alternatively the controller, if the chakra is overactive.

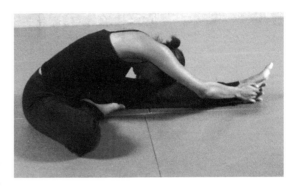

Root Chakra – bent leg forward bend.

1. Assume the plank position from supine by first pressing down on the hands below the shoulders and then raising the chest so that the body is aligned from the heels to the shoulders. Keep the legs extended.
2. Sit cross-legged or in lotus with hands palms down on the knee.
3. Visualize the colour yellow. Inhale and on the exhalation sound 'ah' as in father.

Heart Chakra

This is located in the centre of the chest and is green with a pink hue. This area deals with unconditional love. It is a strong healing energy, but if undernourished can result in loss of self-esteem, and if overactive can result in ego tripping. Body parts are arms, hands and heart.

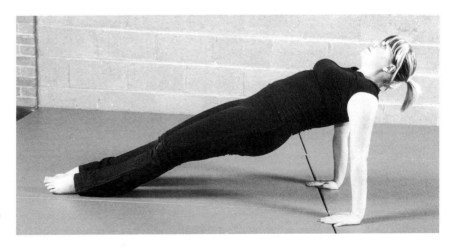

Solar plexus chakra – the plank.

1. Sit cross-legged and extend arms out stretching behind to open up the chest area. Breathe deeply.
2. Place the right hand across the chest on your left shoulder and the left hand on the right shoulder.
3. Close your eyes and be with the colour green. Inhale and on the exhalation sound 'ay' as in play.

Throat Chakra

This is located in the middle of the throat and is blue. This area is associated with communication, not just in a verbal or literal sense but linked with all creative expression and intuition. This chakra is one of the upper areas that is affected by the balance of the lower chakras. Corresponding body parts are the throat, neck, shoulders and lungs.

1. Assume the plough position using the support where necessary as shown previously in this chapter.
2. Return to crossed-legged and visualize the colour blue. Inhale and on the exhalation sound an 'ee' as in teeth.

Brow Chakra

This is located in the middle of the brow and is often called the third eye, being connected to our ability to see or understand the world clearly and with our powers of analysis. The colour is either indigo or silver and it corresponds to the eye and brain.

1. Sit cross-legged and keeping in a seated position, place the hands behind the body so as to extend the chest and take the head upwards. Take the attention to the brow centre and breathe.
2. Return to sitting and place the hands on the knees with the palms upward and the index finger touching the thumb. This is the *mudra* or hand position that represents the union of the individual (index finger) with the universal (thumb).
3. Take a few moments to visualize indigo, then inhale and on the exhalation make the sound 'om'. Now you have done the most infamous and much mocked of all yoga poses – but with an insight into its purpose!

Crown Chakra

This is located at the top of the spine and is our connection with the cosmic world. It is either deep violet or gold in colour. It is our spiritual centre and is linked with enlightenment. The energy in this area develops with maturity, wisdom and independence. The asana for this is the headstand (king of postures) or the preparation for headstand (rabbit pose).

1. Work on a mat or blanket. Kneel down and place your hands on the floor either by (a) having your palms flat on the floor or (b) by clasping your hands together and placing your forearms on the floor in the shape of a triangle.
2. Place your head on the floor either (a) above your palms making a triangle shape, or (b) in between your elbows at the bottom of the triangle.
3. Bring your hips in line with your head so that you have a straight back. You will need to walk your feet towards your body to get some height in the torso. Stay in this position if you do not feel confident to continue. *Only proceed to the full headstand if you are practised in this position or have a teacher to help you.*
4. You may do this against a wall to build confidence. Establish a strong base triangle of hands and head so that you can slowly lift the legs off the ground. Bend your knees and establish your stability before raising them to the extended position. You may take one leg at a time. Take your time over this and feel the energy circulating rather than rushing into it, which can cause you to feel dizzy. Breathe.
5. Lower the legs onto the floor so that the lower legs are rested and you can come up to kneeling.
6. Sit crossed-legged visualizing violet or gold. Inhale and on the exhalation sound 'ng' as in sing.

Chakras in Performance

An understanding of the chakra system is invaluable for performers, enabling them to identify and rebalance their own body energies. Indeed, there are specialist voice teachers who work extensively with mantras to unlock chakras and develop and extend vocal potential. Musicians find the work helpful in order to connect with the rhythms and qualities of each chakra, for example the earthy tribal sounds of the base chakra or the lyricism of the heart. Energizing the chakras can also be useful in performance, whether in work directly connected with character essences or in tuning into the mood of a piece. So, work on the base chakra can be helpful for solid, grounded types whilst the ambitious character can lead from the solar plexus energy and the noble character from the heart. For nurturing roles, the sacrum can be accessed, for communicative characters the throat, and for analytical roles, the energy can be led by the brow centre.

As with the *Five Elements*, there are obviously aspects of these qualities in all of us but we might be aware of strong tendencies in one area. Equally, on a physical level we may be aware of weaknesses that tend to manifest themselves when our resources are low. You may be prone to sore throats, or stomach problems that may give an indication as to where there may be stuck energy. It is important to know your own body so that having deliberately stimulated a chakra for the purposes of a performance, you can take steps to rebalance as you wind down afterwards.

Winding Down

After engaging in energy work, you may find yourself buzzing. This is a vulnerable state to be in and you should always take care to reground by first closing down the chakras. This can be done as a simple, sitting visualization focusing on each area in turn from the crown to the root. Imagine the chakra as an open flower that is now closing up its petals. Alternatively, imagine the light of energy that is slowly dimming until it is a pinprick. Other positions that calm the chakras are either the Child pose (*see* Chapter 3) or the traditional yoga relaxation pose, *Savasana*.

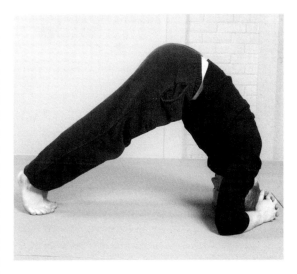

Crown chakra – alternative headstand position.

Savasana – The Classic Yoga Relaxation Asana

1. Lie on the floor with legs extended and arms by the side, allowing the palms to face upward, accepting energy. Close your eyes.
2. Breathe deeply and surrender to the floor.
3. Dissolve any residual areas of tension by breathing through them.
4. You may begin to be aware of the body feeling both heavy as it sinks into the floor and yet light with the sense of energy present in the body.
5. Let the mind be still, just focusing gently on the rise and fall of the breath.

Stand and ground yourself by walking slowly around the room, feeling the earth beneath your feet. Really notice your surroundings, allowing your eyes to be wide and clear as you reconnect with the world.

Throughout the chapter, energy has been sourced through breathing, stretching, sounding, visualizing and touching. Often when feeling a little jaded we try to push ourselves to be energetic but using a more holistic approach, we can get more effective results by tapping into the body's natural channels.

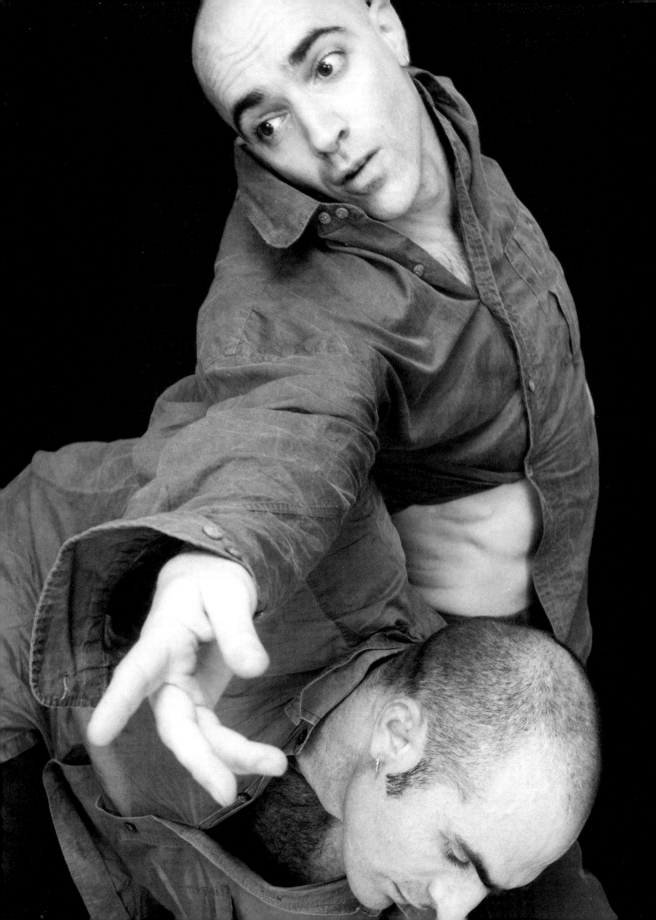

5 DISORIENTATION

Generally speaking, we tend to think about disorientation as being an undesirable place to be, one we might not choose to enter willingly unless we're drunk or in love. To many it will hold negative connotations that signify being in some way out of control. Expressions such as 'giddy', 'head over heels in love', or 'feet don't touch the ground' can feel reckless and somehow irresponsible. Sometimes, we do things when we are feeling disorientated that we might later regret. However, the state of vulnerability that we associate with disorientation can sometimes benefit creativity since it forces us to act from a slightly different place from where we normally operate, a place outside our comfort zone. It is likely that in this state of unknowing we are able to draw on reserves from deep inside

ourselves and get beyond predictable responses. It is through the very experience of physical disorientation that the mind is able to see the world afresh and may be able to respond to it with a renewed sense of creativity.

So much of our daily movement tends to be upright and centred on the forward plane, straight in front of our eyes. In this chapter, we will explore a variety of activities that aim to take us off balance and deny our habitual reliance on our eyes, so that we lose our footing and are forced to respond instead in more instinctive ways. The exercises help to build up trust in our ability to cope with the unexpected and a sense of being able to take risks and respond 'in the moment' to a stimulus. Many of them test our ability to really listen to ourselves and to those around us, drawing

Seeing the world from a different place.

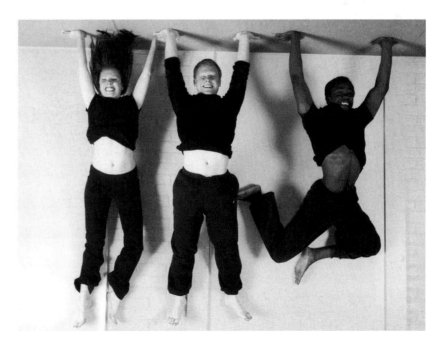

OPPOSITE: *Russell Maliphant company engaged in contact improvisation.*
Photograph by Hugo Glendinning

on neglected senses other than sight. Very often what checks our sense of adventure is fear. As seen in Chapter 3, the wood element is connected with adventure, whilst water is connected with fear. Instead of being petrified, we need to soften our bodies and go with the flow. Exploring the water element helps us break down our fears by encouraging us to glide, surf and dissolve resistances. Revisit the work on the Five Elements Tai Chi work and 'surf' in the water element to prepare yourself for disorientation. Or make a wobble board by placing a board or tray on a hard ball and trying to balance. See how you need to soften your limbs and shift your weight around the centre in order to stop yourself from falling. Disorientation is about adapting to changes occurring underfoot by staying grounded.

Courage, Sensitivity and Trust

Part of the trick of benefiting from disorientation is to get a feel for how to trust oneself and one's surroundings. One of the things we notice about children is how in spite of engaging in apparently reckless activities and launching with enthusiasm into the unknown, they generally emerge from their adventures unscathed. It's partly because the relaxed body is a soft body and one that bounces rather than breaks. As we get older, we tend to tense up to protect ourselves against mishaps and loss of dignity and so we may already be in a state of 'guarding' before the unexpected has occurred. We have only to think about the act of falling, something that children do every day and yet rarely come to grief over. As grown ups it's a much harder thing to fall without getting hurt even if that hurt is only to our pride.

Before throwing ourselves onto potentially dangerous ground, we begin with preliminary exercises and activities drawn from a variety of sources that help us to regain a sense of trust in others and the world around us through a sensitized process of 'letting go'. We then go on to consider the practice of Contact Improvisation and to work practically with the benefits of disorientation offered by this movement form, whose roots lie in the eastern disciplines of tai chi, judo and aikido. Potentially, all the experiences offered in this chapter give the feeling of passing through danger to safety, or of a challenge or risk that's been successfully negotiated. Fearful people frequently feel a sense of satisfaction at having overcome a dread of passing through the unknown, emerging with an increased trust in both themselves and others and a sense of empowerment. Dare-devils however, often need to regain their balance and connect with others by becoming sensitive to the trust placed in them. Risky exercises requiring particular caution are signalled in the text. These should only be attempted by more experienced physical performers.

Wakame

This is a Japanese word for sea anemone, or the kind of seaweed that grows upwards from the seabed and floats up towards the surface of the water. Use soft, lyrical music with unexpected changes of rhythm. In this solo exercise, you need to get a clear sense of your feet being rooted to the ground, like the underwater roots of the plant, but all above the seabed floats freely. This firm, but not static, contact of the feet into the ground allows the rest of the body to swirl from the ankles upwards as the joints become very soft and free. Making sure your eyes are closed, allow the limbs, torso and head to move around in the currents of an imaginary ocean. You will probably shift your weight around, behind and above you. Notice your body spiralling and twisting in different directions as the joints tug and swirl in the underwater ebb and flow.

Granite and Feathers

This is an exercise to do with resistance and letting go. The attention is very much focused in the hara.

1. Half the group lie on the ground and feel as heavy as granite rocks, keeping the hara low and firm. The other half try to pick them up. Notice how hard this is – you may not even be able to do it.
2. Now the granite group imagines being feather-weight instead of rock-like. The sensation in the hara is of lightness and elevation. Partners just guide their movements upwards from the

Pendulum swing.

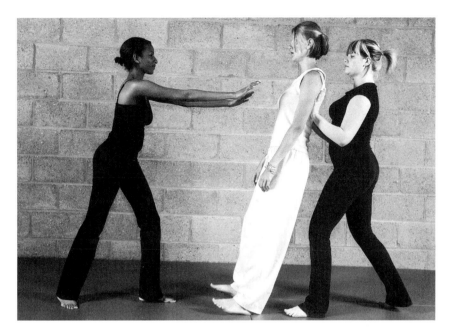

floor and this time they will rise up in a very different way, like the wind lifting up a feather.

You will discover that very rigid, resistant bodies are hard to shift. A soft, yielding body will move with ease.

Pendulum Swing
This is the classic trust exercise that can be very revealing of the extent to which someone is prepared to *trust* themselves to the care and support of their partners. Some people will find it easy to trust the supporting partners, especially if the supporters are quite strong looking. For others, the exercise can be a real challenge and in some cases quite an ordeal. Be sensitive and build up the trust slowly by not standing too far away from the mover until they feel more at ease.

Two people stand facing one another, at least a metre apart with one foot placed forwards and the other behind, to stabilize. A third (who will be rocked between the others) stands between them, feet slightly apart.

1. Everybody breathes and allows the neck to be soft. The person on the inside is rocked between the two outer people who support at the shoulders and upper chest. Make sure that the supporters keep a firm contact with the ground and keep their knees bent with the centre of gravity low. Build up the rocking rhythm very slowly, like a pendulum, straight but not stiff.

2. The supporting partners need to make sure that they do not halt the movement, but catch it like a ball: absorb the movement by continuing it and then pushing it back in the opposite direction.

3. The person being rocked needs to think of their body as being in a long line, so try not to collapse in the centre by bending too much at the waist or knee. When the momentum and contact are moving well, the supporters can take a step apart, slowly extending the distance between them; receive on the in-breath, push away on the exhalation. Everyone breathe through the feet and this will really help with the trust and elasticity.

Falling Around the Circle
(More advanced version of above exercise)
This needs to be done in a group, preferably with about six or eight people. Ideally, you should all have had first-hand experience of the two previous exercises.

1. Form a circle facing inwards with one person in the centre. Those around the edge get quite close together and take one foot back to support themselves, keeping the centre of gravity low as in the previous exercise.
2. The person in the centre begins to gently sway towards the circle. As they do so, their weight is supported on their upper chest and shoulder area by the hands of the group members. The weight of the centre person can be quite heavy, so make sure that as many people as possible make contact to support them. As in the pendulum swing exercise, the centre person needs to feel soft enough to give their body weight to the supporters, but not so collapsed as to fall down into a heap.
3. As the centre person gains confidence, they are able to give more and more of their weight. A very released person may even begin to turn full circles. It is a very powerful exercise that challenges some people, but one that can be profoundly liberating once the body gives permission to let go.

You should now feel soft and free enough to attempt the following 'falling' exercise that requires a real sense of controlled release.

Falling to the Ground Like Silk
Take a silk scarf, throw it into the air and observe how it wafts down towards the ground, gently folding itself in. Bear this image in mind as you try the following exercise. Start on a mat first to build confidence.

1. Walk around taking deep, soft breaths.
2. Soften the neck and other joints and on an exhalation, allow yourself to sink to the ground by just letting go of all your resistances. Having a sensation of yourself as silk, allow yourself to unravel downwards.
3. It's a good idea to think of yourself falling sideways allowing your calves to cushion you, rather than trying rigidly to drop forward onto the knees.

When you first try this exercise it feels anything but silky: the body may be quite stiff and clumsy. As you continue, you will gain confidence and the whole falling process will feel possible, and even pleasurable.

Slithering Down Partner's Body
Approach this exercise by building up through a number of stages.

1. One person stands rooted, strong and with a low centre of gravity.
2. The second person begins by wrapping themselves around their supporter, using either arm(s) or leg(s) to make good contact and leaning their weight into the body of the standing person.
3. Tune into the breathing pattern of your partner by sensing the movement of your partner's ribcage and on a mutual exhalation, find a way of sliding down your partner's body to the floor, keeping contact until the last moment, when you roll away.
4. Try this several times and swap over.
5. When you are comfortable with this exercise you can try just leaning and sliding down without the preliminary wrapping of limbs.

Catch Me!
This, potentially risky exercise should only be attempted when you feel confident with the previous exercises. Again, you can experience this in several stages.

1. Begin in pairs standing one in front of the other. The person in front leans their weight back onto the body of supporting partner behind who then 'catches' them lowering them gently to the ground. The supporter is not 'carrying' the weight of their partner but using gravity to absorb the force and ease them to the floor. Try this several times and swap over.

You can then proceed to the more advanced version that is basically the same thing but performed with movement in between that gives a different dynamic to the exercise. Be very aware of safety – the position of the catcher must be grounded and centred. Keep a long spine and soft neck, bending your knees as you lower your partner to the ground.

1. Four or more people in a large space, preferably one with carpets or mats, jog slowly around. Change directions when you feel like it.
2. At a certain point, someone taps the person in front on the shoulder. This is the cue for them to allow their weight to fall backwards into the receiving arms of the tapper.
3. The receiver needs to support by having a strong hara and positioning one leg slightly behind them. Let the person fall back onto your body and take them to the floor by allowing them to drop gently over to the side where your back foot is located. They will then continue the momentum of the fall by rolling over and standing up: both set off at a slow jog again.
4. Keep tapping and falling whilst building up the pace.

Glass Cobra

This is a famous Augusto Boal exercise that develops the senses and builds intimacy and connection between group members. It involves initial contact with a partner whom you then lose only to seek them out again. The process of recovering them creates the need for a disorientating quest in which you only have your sense of touch to guide you!

Six or eight is a good group size, working on a carpet or matted area as the exercise may involve some crawling.

1. Group stands in a circle, each facing clockwise with eyes closed. Group leader then mixes up the positions by taking people out and re-organizing them so that they are standing in front of somebody different.
2. Each person now takes time to feel the head, neck and shoulders of the person in front. Even sniff to see if there is a distinctive odour. You should really be sensitive to the uniqueness of your partner. Give them a gentle massage on neck and shoulders, even extending to the upper arms.

3. Group leader then separates the whole group by leading the members individually to different parts of the room. Each person then kneels.
4. When the leader gives the signal, set off in quest of your partner. You will need to crawl your way very gingerly until you reach another person. When you do, feel whether this is your partner or not. If not, pass on.
5. If, however, you have now formed part of the link of the snake, stay with them and move together in quest of their front half and so on until all the pieces of the cobra are put together again. When the chain is complete, there should be a great sense of being reunited and back home again after a feeling of frag-mentation and loss.

Trusting to the Structures

In creating an environment in which we are prepared to lose control, we must make sure that there is a safety net to catch us when we fall. We get support not only from our partners but also from structures around us, the most important of which is the floor. In previous chapters we have seen how the earth allows us to surrender to gravity. So make a friend of the floor. As partners offering support we also need a real sense, with grounded bodies, of the earth beneath us. We can learn from certain physical positions that are low in their centre of gravity offering strong bases to support the disorientated partner: stone, table,

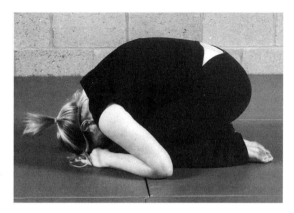

Stone.

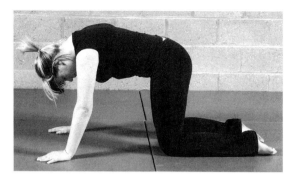

Table.

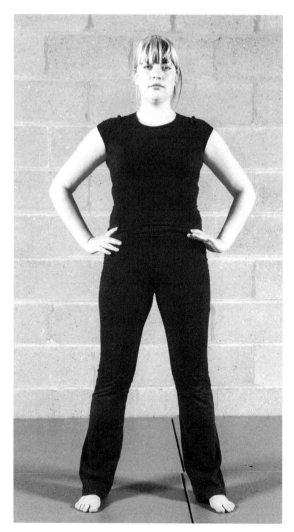

Tree.

tree. Experiment around your partner's stable base in these three positions to find ways in which you can use this support to balance. Proceed with caution – be aware that the waist area in 'table' is a weak area of the back as it has no ribcage protecting the vital organs.

Leaping

Whilst the preceding exercises have encouraged in us a sense of falling and embracing the earth, we can also use this stable contact with the ground to encourage elevation.

1. Take a run towards a wall and leap up to reach a spot as high as you can. Instinctively you will reach out with the other hand to touch the wall to protect your body from hitting it. Be aware of this and try to take that hand a little higher each time in order to encourage the reaching hand to extend further. It will feel a little like climbing a ladder.
2. Advanced students may want to explore the possibilities of leaping and reaching by using their partner in either the stone, table or tree positions to achieve even more height. (Warning: this is potentially risky – you should aim to use the sacrum, thighs and interlinked hands.)
3. Begin at the wall and then explore the possibilities of working beyond the safety of the vertical support.

Raising the Body

Group exercise. Minimum of eight people. Use mats or a padded floor surface.

This is an initially daunting exercise that when executed with co-ordinated attention by the supporters, gives the 'rider' a miraculous sense of weightlessness and freedom that is very liberating.

1. The person who is going to be lifted starts stretched out on the floor on their back with their eyes closed.
2. The rest of the group space themselves out and kneel beside them with one knee up, placing their palms under the prone body. Remember to give extra support at the head and the hips, these being the heaviest parts of the body.

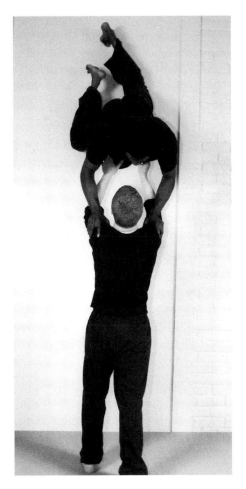 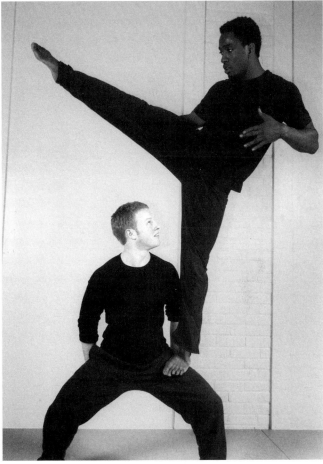

Using the wall.   *Launching from the tree.*

3. On the count of three, the group comes to standing, gently raising the body off the ground. Keep the knees bent and the spine long, being careful not to strain the back. Stay supporting for a little while so that the person being lifted can have a full sensation of being held.
4. Swap over, changing the positions so every one has a turn at the heaviest end.

Playful Disorientation

It's sometimes very difficult to feel comfortable with intimate bodywork when this is so often associated with sexual contact. Fun exercises can provide a way into a strong sense of physical intimacy that can develop a more sensitive approach to performance interaction. These exercises provide a useful preliminary to the extended work on Contact Improvisation in which the slightest body contact activates an impulse. This has an important application to the wider sense of performance since, even when no physical contact occurs on stage, there is a need to respond to the invisible currents of energy. We need to detect the subtle impulses sent out by fellow performers and be able to respond spontaneously with each fresh performance. In the very process of disorientation, we experience a heightened sense of the exchange of energy and learn to connect with the give and take of interaction.

Tennis Ball Jazz

In pairs, stand opposite one another and place a soft tennis ball or juggling ball between your foreheads. Dance to a variety of music from Madonna to Mozart. Try and be as loose and rhythmic in your movements as possible whilst keeping the ball in place. If you get very confident with this exercise, try shifting the feet through actual steps and see if you can travel with the ball.

Pony-Riding

For this you need a large clear space since it is potentially hazardous. If you are in a big group, split into two and let one half of the group watch. You need music to trot to – a firm rhythm but not too fast.

1. Take a partner and stand next to them, on their left side. Spend a few minutes massaging their upper back and neck and generally warming up the area. Then take their left hand in yours. Place your right hand on the back of their neck. This is your steering rein. Remember that this is the key area in the Alexander Technique that we need to keep relaxed. Make a good connection with this place, lightly contacting but not pinching.
2. When the music starts, begin to walk with your pony and at this point they close their eyes. Get into a good walking rhythm. Check out how they are responding to the task and be careful to steer them well clear of any other 'ponies' coming your way. This is a very revealing exercise: some people will be really in tune with their partners and raring to go, while others will hold back and may even draw back their heads in trepidation.
3. Only if and when your pony has achieved confident walking, try and take them into a trot. Aim to keep perfectly in step, move as a team. The pony should be easy in its movements and not grimace in apprehension of a crash.
4. Any really connected pony pair can try lifting their knees so that their trots become more spectacular.
5. Swap over and see if a trusting and confident pony is also a good rider.

Initially, this can be a highly disorienting exercise until ponies have relaxed and tuned into the rhythm of their riders. It is up to the rider to slowly give them confidence by careful steering and familiarity. The humour generated by this exercise aids the relaxation process by helping us have fun and not take ourselves too seriously, as in the following exercise.

Leg-Waggling

Cover the floor space with mats. Work in threes, one person lying on the floor.

1. Second and third people stand, one at the head, and one at the feet end of the person lying down, lifting the person's arms and legs. This is where the fun begins as the standing partners simultaneously begin waggling the limbs of person one. This involves them in raising, then lowering the arms and legs in a quick, successive rhythm. Be playful but sensitive and avoid pulling harshly or wrenching the limbs of the person whose body you are moving. The movement may well bring the hips and shoulders into a rocking movement and the combined action of the people at each end generally has the effect of making the person lying down giggle!
2. If the person agrees and you have enough matting to make this safe, you can then try swinging the person from side to side, holding wrists and ankles and lifting them just clear of the floor as you swing the body from side to side.
3. Some people love the experience of helplessness that this exercise induces. It's also a good feeling to arrive on terra firma again after losing your bearings.

Bareback 'Riding'

One 'rider' and three to five supporters. Thick mats. Not to be undertaken by anyone with a weak back.

1. The supporters line up on all fours, positioning their bodies closely side by side.
2. The 'rider' carefully lowers himself/herself at right angles across the backs of the supporters

ending up lying outstretched with their feet off the ground.

3. Once the 'rider' is securely in position, the supporters begin to arch and release their backs giving the person lying above an undulating ride.

Having completed these preliminary trust and release exercises, we are ready to move on to the main practice.

Contact Improvisation

Contact Improvisation was developed primarily by a dancer called Steve Paxton in America in the 1970s. The form involves a deep sensitization of the body that leads us into some powerfully disorienting states from which we return braver and far more capable of both yielding and giving support when necessary, qualities that can be enormously beneficial to the performer. Paxton originally trained as a gymnast but was also interested in martial arts, specifically aikido. One of his stimuli was an interest in therapeutic movement work with sighted and non-sighted participants. He evolved Contact Improvisation by developing

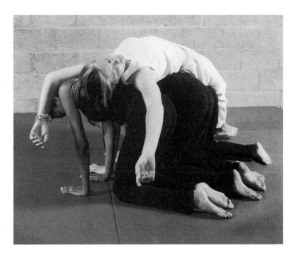

Bareback riding.

the use of contact, breath, gravity, the exchange of weight and the flow of energy between partners. Contact Improvisation may involve leaning, gliding, rolling and slithering over and under your partner in ways that are infinitely surprising. Contact is a highly democratic movement practice that values bodies of all shapes, sizes and capacities and is therefore used extensively in community and therapeutic work as well as in performance. Sometimes it involves both, as in the groundbreaking work of companies like Candoco whose members are drawn from both disabled and able-bodied people mutually supporting one another.

You will notice that many of the exercises described in Contact Work appear to be rather obvious and yet are accompanied by quite detailed explanations. This is because this work is very much about feeling the process and working internally with the quality of the movement exchange. In this respect, it can feel much like Feldenkrais. Avoid the temptation to race through these exercises performing them in an external way, as this will only lead to a mechanical response and you will miss out on the holistic benefits.

The Benefits of Contact Improvisation for Performers Include:

- Developing qualities of trust, support and listening (kinaesthetically) to a partner – cardinal qualities needed for successful performance.
- Sensitizing participants to the *process* rather than the product.
- Encouraging spontaneity as movements evolve naturally from the dancer's moment-by-moment choices.
- Developing the performer's holistic awareness of themselves and others.
- Encourages an exhilarating sense of disorientation that can only be reached through a state of relaxed attentiveness.
- Develops the performer's somatic sense through an awareness of inner spaces and feeling through the skin.

Lying Down Prior to Contact Work

One of the founders of Contact Improvisation, Steve Paxton laid great emphasis on the value of lying down as a preliminary to contact work. He believed that in a modern world that was fast-paced, multifocused and frequently unreliable, enormous stability was to be gained from letting go our resistances and simply trusting to the floor to earth us and bear our weight. Until you have learned to trust gravity to support you, there is little chance that you will be able to either give or take weight effectively with a partner.

1. Lie in supine on a mat or blanket, paying attention to the length and symmetry.
2. Observe the way your body makes contact with the ground and notice if you're holding your muscles away from the ground or allowing the joints to sink naturally. Imagine your body sinking to meet the floor.
3. If you feel yourself holding on, particularly in the hips, lower back and shoulders, consciously breathe into the area and try to soften and release, allowing your weight to come into greater contact with the ground at each exhalation. As Paxton reminds us, when lying down, the fundamental consideration is the existence of the floor, your body and the surface between them where they meet. By focusing on this and ridding the mind of extraneous thoughts, we will achieve a better quality of contact and release with the ground.

At this point, any of the Feldenkrais sequences from Chapter 2 would be excellent as preparation for the partner work in Contact Improvisation. Feldenkrais work encourages an extraordinary sensation of giving weight to and being supported by the ground as you slowly roll and release through the infinitesimal movements. Moreover, very often in Feldenkrais work we are not quite sure of where the movement is taking us next and there is often a feeling that the body is 'falling' into the unknown, a prospect that is potentially scary but liberating. Before we encounter Contact in a full-bodied way, here is a Tai Chi exercise to help sensitize you to your own and your partner's movement impulses. Many of the principles of Tai Chi relate naturally to concepts embodied in Contact work.

Lotus Movement with Partner
This exercise helps you and your partner tune into an 'invisible' connection, drawing on the yin/yang exchange. Your rising arm is the yang energy and as your other arm moves towards the earth, this is the yin energy. In this exercise the forces of yin and yang are in a state of dynamic equilibrium both in your own body and between yourself and your partner. This is a fundamental concept in Contact work, depending as it does, on the flow of give and take between two people.

1. Stand facing your partner far enough apart for you to extend your arms towards each other, with soft elbows, fingertips almost touching.
2. Each of you places one palm facing upwards and the other palm facing downwards and you almost touch fingertips with your partner. Upturned hands should form one pair and downward turned hands the other.
3. Take a breath and slowly release the exhalation as the downward turned pair rises and the upturned pair of hands descend until both pairs of arms are long and fully extended, but not rigid.
4. The movements should be slow and rhythmic and released on the breath as the pairs of hands arrive at both the top and the bottom of the movement simultaneously.
5. Inhale again as you slowly rotate both pairs of hands and begin the ascent/descent reversing the movement on the exhalation and paying special attention to the sensation of hands turning over. As you do so, you simultaneously experience the yin energy transforming to yang, and vice versa.
6. Continue the movements and after a while you can become more playful, perhaps changing the arc of the movement onto the oblique, or lengthening and shortening the distance between the hands when you turn the movements around. Keep your joints light and free, especially your shoulders. Allow your torso to gently rotate and keep the knees and neck soft, and the movements will take you into all sorts of surprising places.

7. Tune into your partner's impulses and sense how far you can mutually explore the possibilities of the basic movements. Don't forget to breathe in as the hands rotate and breathe out on the travelling movements.

Pushing Hands

This is a very important exercise in Tai Chi developing an acutely sensitized contact between partners and quick responsiveness. It is a valuable way to prepare for contact work especially since it encourages a sense of playful inventiveness and 'going with the flow'. It can be very disorienting until one has learned to return to one's centre and not to stiffen up when someone gives you a lot of weight that threatens to throw you off balance. This is a great way of surrendering the ego.

1. Stand opposite your partner, one foot forward, one behind, for stability. Decide who is to begin by 'pushing hands'.
2. This person leads the movement by pushing their hands into the upper chest and the shoulders of their partner who receives and dodges the force by shifting their upper body, from the feet upwards, in such a way as to avoid being toppled over or pushed off their axis.
3. At first this seems impossible but if you keep light limbs and allow the body to shift to the side before returning to the centre, you will get the feel of how to do this. Keep the shoulders relaxed.
4. It's helpful to think of your centre of gravity as low and the movements coming not from the chest, but instead from the *hara*.
5. Imagine you have a pole running down your spine and to the ground, leaning slightly forwards. If you are pushed sideways, bend the knees, and rotate on the axis of that pole but maintain the same slight tilt in the body. Don't be afraid to change the position of your feet if you need to realign yourself. Send the weight back and down through your feet making a small elliptical curve of your body, before rebounding to the centre. You will soon find yourself ducking and weaving but you will always bob up again around your centre.

6. 'Pushing hands' is an activity that can go on for hours as you become increasingly flexible and able to 'get out of a corner'.

At first there will be one distinct leader or 'pusher'. Eventually, when you are a bit more experienced, it is possible to perform this exercise with both people engaged in the push/pull, yin/yang exchange as you work together, alternating the initiating movements; 'Pushing Hands' is just another way of exploring the Tai Chi curve using a dynamic partner exercise that encourages letting go and returning to your centre. It's an ideal preparation for Contact Improvisation, developing both sensitivity and inventiveness.

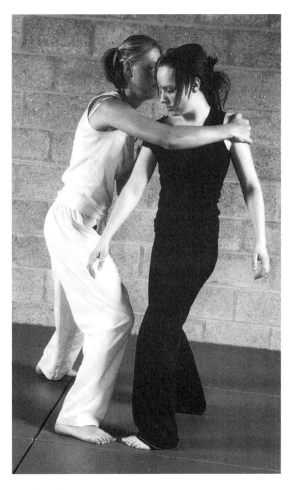

Pushing hands.

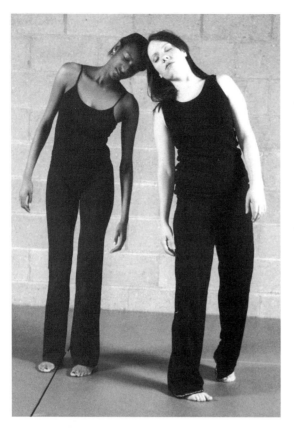

The small dance.

Head to Head Contact Work – Paxton's 'Small Dance'

This is one of Steve Paxton's initial contact exercises that carries within it the essence of the practice.

1. Stand facing your partner, a little way away so that you are leaning slightly inwards and can touch head to head.
2. Touch forehead to forehead. Breathe and give a little pressure to your partner so that you are conscious of the contact between you. The idea is not to ram or head-butt. Neither should you be so passive that you cannot register any sensation in this spot. Maintain a sense of an exchange occurring at the point of contact. Ideally there should be a very small movement as you begin to have a dialogue just through

this point. Keep this going for some time, maybe offering and receiving a little more weight as you go on. At this stage, the idea is not to go anywhere but just to explore the exchange of tiny movements you are generating.

3. Now you can increase the movement and maybe very softly allow your heads to roll around each other by moving your ears together, then taking the movement back through the forehead and to the other side. Really feel the implications of the movement through the weight distribution of the rest of the body shifting to accommodate the change of position.
4. Eventually, when you are practised at doing this, try rolling around the whole head and luxuriate in the feeling of giving weight through the back of the head. This will probably involve your back, neck and shoulders in a releasing peeling off action.
5. You can experiment around this interaction with a variety of other body parts such as shoulders, or hips. The trick is always to keep the movements very slow and 'felt'. Breathing is very important to connect and sensitize you to your partner's impulses.

Once you have got the feel of rolling around various common body parts you can be more explorative and trace unbroken pathways around the body surface using a variety of different body parts. This process is known as 'mapping the body'.

'Flying' with a Partner

This is a liberating exercise requiring a highly responsive yet relaxed contact with your partner. If performed with tension or fear it can become hard work and will be unrewarding. Lyrical music helps the flow of the contact.

1. Stand behind your partner and give their shoulders a brief massage.
2. Slip your arms underneath theirs – tune into each other's breathing patterns.
3. On an exhalation slowly allow your partner's arms to float up. You will now be lightly supporting their limbs but don't allow any tension to creep in.

4. As always, keep necks, hips and knees free and released.

5. Begin to move, exploring the space all around you, above, to the sides and in front. Use your arms to both explore and to counterbalance.

6. Allow the arms to unfold and fold again as the joints and the torso move freely. It's as if you are both sharing gigantic wings. This exercise really encourages some luxuriant counter-pointed rhythms with limbs and joints in free flow.

7. Breathe freely and if you feel yourself stiffening or becoming heavy, return to small, light movements. The sensation should be of gliding weightlessly. Try to re-create the sensation of the seaweed exercise (Wakame) at the beginning of Chapter 5.

Rocking the Bones

This begins as a gentle manipulation and develops into some fluid rolling and releasing movements. Use padded mats. Work in pairs.

1. Your partner lies in supine with their eyes closed.

2. Kneel at their side and using two hands gently rock their bones by making small rolling movements. One leg at a time, start at the ankles and work your way up the shins making a movement similar to rolling pastry – never pressing down but allowing the muscles to spread with the rolling action. Really feel for the bones with your palms and connect with the ground beneath. You can work the joints, but be very gentle in areas like the knees and elbows.

3. The person being rocked needs to surrender themselves to the rocking movements and not resist or tighten up. Feel the joints loosen and enjoy the sensation of the muscle releasing from the bones. The rocker starts with small movements and builds it up to be slightly more vigorous once the muscles feel relaxed and the joints begin to release.

4. Once you have worked your way up both legs, kneeling at the side of the body, place your palms on either hip bone and rock them back and forth, feeling the pelvis making contact

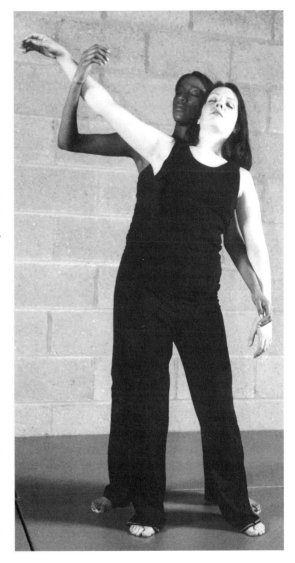

Flying with a partner.

with the floor for stability. Take the rocking action to the ribcage.

5. Now move to the arms and starting at the wrists work up the bones. You should take your time over this exercise so that the whole rocking sequence lasts for at least ten minutes. Ensure that you are relaxed in the movement and that your spine is long so that you do not transmit any tension to your partner.

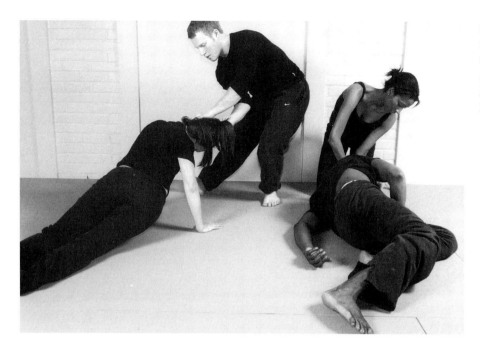

Supported movement from the floor, developing from Rocking the Bones.

Stage Two – Extending to Movement

6. Now turn your partner from their back onto their side. This can be done quite easily by lifting the knee closest to you into the semi-supine position. Place one hand just below the knee and the other hand at the hip and move the leg over to their opposite side in an upwards direction to bring them into position. Bring the arm over to join the leg.

7. Continue with the rocking action on the side of the body but this time just gently engage the fingertips so that the impulse is taken on by your partner. They should feel a response to the tidal wave of movement and allow their body to release and return (notice the similarities to Feldenkrais). Being in side position enables a greater freedom of movement as the spine is free to respond to the impulse.

8. Keep a light rolling contact as your partner begins to initiate their own rhythms and personal movement signature that may involve moments of rest or stillness. You might encourage them to eventually roll right over or move through to a sitting position.

9. Conclude by returning through the movements to lying, and then to the initial sensitive 'rocking the bones' and so to stillness.

Head Supported Movement
The following pair exercise is best done following the Neck Jazz exercise given in Chapter 1.

1. One person lies in supine and the other places their hands gently on the sides of their partner's head, making light cradling contact.

2. Both partners breathe and tune in to each other as the person lying down is encouraged by the hands on their head to begin to create their own small movements, starting with the head and eventually letting the movement flow into the upper body and then the arms.

3. Do not hurry but allow the movement to develop according to your own internal rhythms and inclinations as your partner responds to the gentle contact of your hands on their head.

4. Eventually the movement will slowly bring you to rise to sit and eventually to stand. Your partner continues to follow the movements until they come to a natural rest. Swap over.

Embracing the Wall

This exercise involves you in a relationship with the floor and a clear wall space.

1. Close your eyes and make contact with the wall. This may involve taking weight on the hands.
2. Think about the journey from wall to floor and back again, allowing your body weight to make contact with the supporting surfaces.
3. At first, your movements will be quite tentative but see how far you can trust yourself to gravity and contact in your exploration of the space around you. See how many different body surfaces you can engage with the wall and the floor in the course of your journey. See how far you can take the body upside down to find interesting weight-bearing travelling positions.

Sightless Exploration of the Space

This group exercise requires a clear space.

1. The group members position themselves around the edges of the room, evenly spaced. All close eyes. Everyone makes contact with a wall and at a given signal, keeping some contact, all begin to move slowly in a clockwise direction.
2. Proceed very slowly to explore the perimeter of the space, rolling and shifting the weight through whatever body part is in contact with the upright surface and the floor.
3. When the group members have travelled around the entire space, give a signal to leave the walls slowly and move into the centre of the room. Move very slowly and be prepared to negotiate other bodies on your journey to the centre. The contact will be very soft and light.
4. When all the members have arrived in the middle, sit with crossed legs and finish in a circle.

Back-to-Back Contact

This is the place from which Contact work often

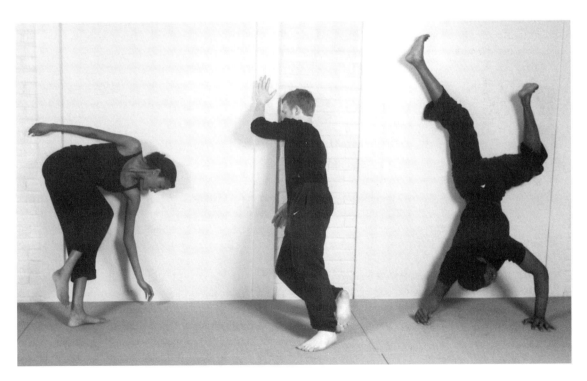

Embracing the wall.

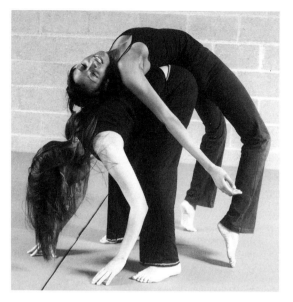

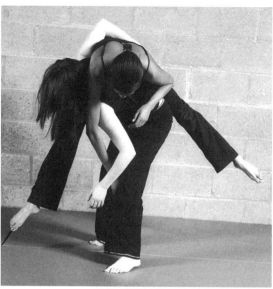

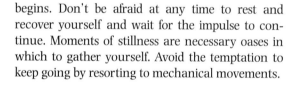

Contact work emerging from back to back.

Contact work in action.

begins. Don't be afraid at any time to rest and recover yourself and wait for the impulse to continue. Moments of stillness are necessary oases in which to gather yourself. Avoid the temptation to keep going by resorting to mechanical movements.

1. Sit back to back with your partner, maybe a little apart at the hips. Begin by making contact on the back of the head and rolling from side to side.
2. Now try taking your head over your partner's shoulder and just giving weight in this position. Enjoy the sensation in your spine and neck as you do so. Spend time in each of these positions and try rolling right across your partner's shoulders as you twist one shoulder forward and your weight away from your partner. There will come a point where you are only connected at the opposite shoulder and now you can reverse the action and roll back bringing the other shoulder towards your partner. This shared contact may even extend through to your arms.
3. Now feel what is going on in your partner's back. Does it feel warm and alive, or cold and dull? Is it lively with sensation or solid? Begin to

experiment with the shoulder blades, now giving weight, now receiving your partner's, sensing when to give weight and when to receive. In order to do this, you will have to allow the left and right sides of your body to move independently. Think of the transfer of weight like a tide rushing in to fill a space.
4. Begin to shift and release the back, not forgetting the possible contact between heads and neck. Consider the possibility of allowing the hips to rise so that you can shift your upper body weight onto the support of your partner's back and vice versa. The only rule is that you should remain in contact with your partner through some body part.
5. At this point, couples often lose the back-to-back contact altogether and take off in a free movement dialogue that may take them away from the ground into lifts and rolls and gliding movements. Don't predict or anticipate movement but respond in the moment: you are not trying to form fixed positions. If the exchange of weight is occurring sensitively, it should feel like giving and receiving an ever-shifting massage, which is why Contact work, besides being exquisite to watch, can be so therapeutic.

Reconnecting to the Earth

The process of *Disorientation* encourages a powerful contact with our *Wood* element taking us off our secure base and on a journey into the unknown. The wood element is deeply associated with the movement of the wind, and you will appreciate the connection to this in the adventurous exercises you have just experienced. The value of the wind impetus is that it encourages us to take risks in spite of ourselves. With such risk-taking, there is often a huge physical and emotional investment that can pay dividends for our creativity. You may have come up against some of your own fears in this work that you may not have completely overcome. This is natural but remember that even in becoming more aware of the nature of our fears there is a potential growth. After such unsettling but potentially exhilarating experiences, it is often valuable to return to the restorative security of the *Earth*. The next chapter looks at the whole process of Grounding through earthing ourselves. In order to prepare for this, we will end with a yoga balancing pose, but first revisit the Child pose, given in Chapter 4.

Tree Pose

After the calming effect of the child pose, the tree pose is very grounding. It can only really be practised to full effect if we think of rooting into the ground beneath us on the standing leg. It can be performed freestanding in the centre of a room, or with our back to a wall to give extra stability.

1. Start on one leg and bending the other leg to the side, lift the foot with your hands and press the sole of the bent leg against the opposite thigh.
2. Really think the standing leg into the ground, spreading the toes out lifting both sides of the ankles evenly.
3. When secure in this position, feel the opening of the hip on the bent leg side. Resist the impulse to let this hip rise up.
4. Lengthen the waist by drawing in the abdomen on the out breath and feeling the lower spine dropping down to the earth. Resist the

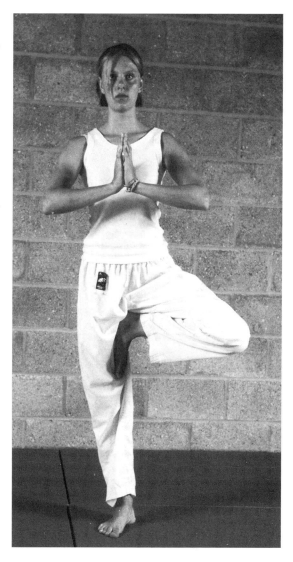

Tree pose with hands in prayer position.

temptation to stick the bottom out. Stay in this position with the hands in prayer.
5. Alternatively, when secure, raise the arms above the head. As you feel the sensation of lifting up through the torso, allow the foot to make strong contact with the ground, keeping the connection with the earth. Relax the face and jaw.
6. Breathe freely and repeat on the other side.

113

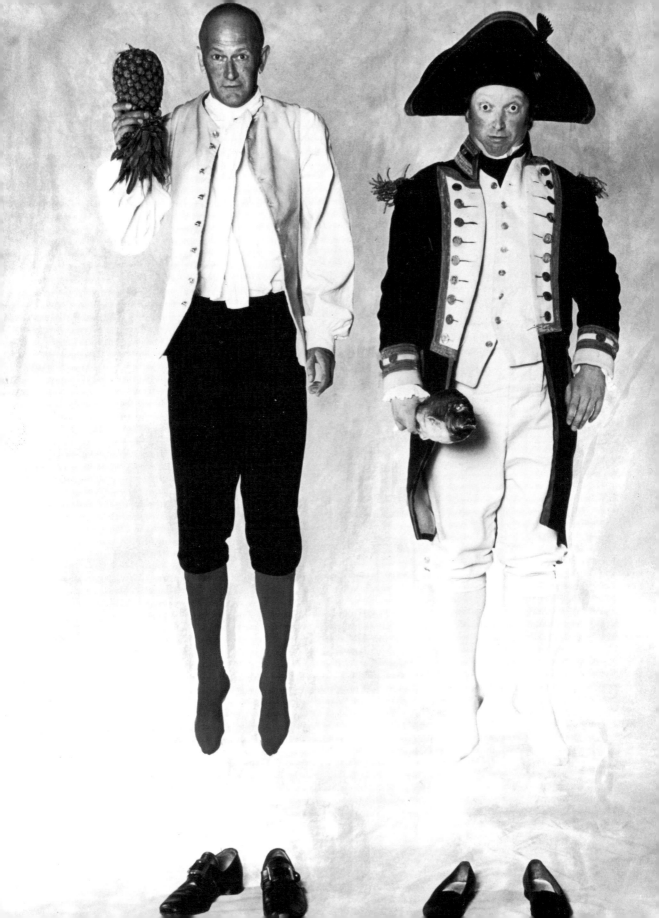

6 GROUNDING

It's no coincidence that the foot is a neglected area of the body. After all, it's at the opposite end from the head that we 'look up to' as the generator of our thinking. Some people feel queasy about the very idea of their feet or anyone else's, as the feet are often where inhibitions are tightly locked. Even dancers, for whom the foot is a primary source of expression, can often regard feet in a purely mechanical way and treat them with disrespect. Every day we give our feet a battering, often forcing them into tight shoes and walking on concrete paving that impacts on the soles sending jolts through the whole body. Yet we forget that our feet are in some ways more sensitive than our hands. Babies first explore the world through their feet and it is to this openness we hope to return by taking off our shoes and connecting with the earth.

There is a great range of cultural traditions associated with the foot, the most famous of which is probably Chinese foot-binding that now holds quite negative gender associations. Yet the power of the feet is celebrated in rituals of fire-walking, where a rite of passage is enacted through walking across hot coals unscathed. The feet can be sites of repression or liberation. Politics, gender, power are all expressed through the choice of footwear and the attendant walks. And it's a fact that many actors base characterizations around observations of shoes and walking. Shoes affect the feet in a physical way, sensualizing them, or distorting their shape, causing all sorts of misalignments in the body. The history of a person is strongly identified by their shoes, which explains how central feet are to the performer's communication.

OPPOSITE: *Told by an Idiot in* **I Can't Wake Up.**
Photograph by Richard Lewisohn

This chapter offers some significant opportunities to work from the foot upwards. The first set of exercises helps you to re-familiarize yourself with your feet and all that they stand for. It takes you through some reflexology and a variety of grounding exercises drawn from yoga and other bodywork practices. A second set of activities helps you recover a sense of playful inventiveness through working with the feet, a skill that's highly relevant for the creative process. The final section explores some possibilities for creative movement in relation to the story of *The Red Shoes.* This is one of the most significant fairy tales that we have concerning feet and the claiming of creative identity. The grounding work in this chapter relates strongly to the Earth element, putting us more fully in contact with our instinctive selves. It is our place of recovery and strength and the centre from which our creativity and balance is nurtured and replenished. By the end of this chapter the expression 'standing on your own two feet' should have a new meaning for you.

REFLEXOLOGY

Reflexology is an ancient practice of healing through touching pressure points in the feet (or hands). The foot is seen to be a perfect map of the whole body and by applying pressure to the various reflex areas of the foot it is possible to make a connection with the body's organs and systems. The nerves work as messengers from the feet sending energy, helping the body rebalance and relieving tension. The reflexologist first uses massage to stimulate and relax the feet and then applies pressure to the reflex areas with a caterpillar walking action. If you get a feel for it by working on your own feet you can actually identify tiny little

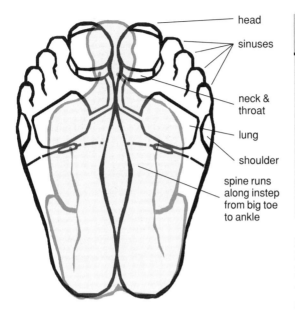

A simplified diagram of foot reflex areas.

head

sinuses

neck & throat

lung

shoulder

spine runs along instep from big toe to ankle

lumps underneath the skin, caused by a build up of uric acid or calcium crystals. The sensation of massaging these crystals is a bit like popping bubble wrap. These may be found in tender spots, often indicating that there has been some tension or imbalance in the referred area.

Contra-indications
Don't treat anyone who is: in early stages of pregnancy, suffering from a blood clot or DVT.

Preparation
First practise caterpillar thumb walking on yourself to get the right pressure. The thumb should not lose contact with the skin between steps – it glides firmly, moving half a centimetre at a time. When you hold the foot, make sure that the fingers on your other hand are providing a counter-support so that you are not digging into your partner's foot, but you can feel the pressure between your own hands.

Get your partner to lie down on a blanket on the floor with both their head and knees raised on pillows. Clean the feet with some wet wipes. Make sure you are comfortably seated at the feet of your partner. It is important that you keep your spine long in this position so either kneel or sit cross-legged with cushions supporting. The reflexologist would normally use a massage bed or specially designed chair to access the feet from a more comfortable position. Rub a little cream or a little baby powder into the feet so that your hands can glide but don't slip over the skin.

A 20-Minute Reflexology Sequence

This sequence has been devised especially with performers in mind since it focuses on the vital areas of the throat, chest, spine and shoulders which all affect breathing and the voice. The sequence is explained for right-handers: reverse instructions for left-handers.

Opening Massage
1. Take your partner's right foot and supporting the ankle with the left hand underneath, rotate the foot with the right hand holding the ball. Start with gentle little circles and then increase these to open the ankle. Rotate in both directions.
2. Two-way stretch. Firmly cradle the underside of the right ankle in your left hand and gently pull it towards you along the Achilles tendon. Then use your right hand to push the ball of the foot away from you. Release and repeat several times.
3. Supporting the foot in your lap, hold the ball of the foot in both hands and squeeze slightly to find the hollow in the sole under the big toe

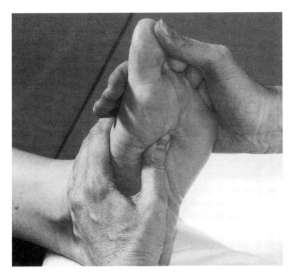

Thumb working solar plexus.

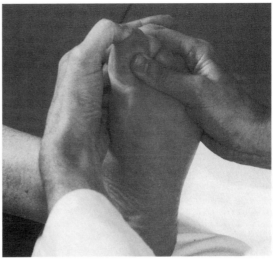

Caterpillar thumb walking over big toe (head).

bulge. Place your thumbs (one on top of the other) into this solar plexus area. Spread your fingers over the front of the foot then draw them back as you apply pressure with the thumbs. This helps to open the chest.

Repeat for left foot.

Pressure Point Sequence
1. Begin by supporting the right toe with your left hand and applying pressure with the right thumb making a caterpillar walking movement around the toe (head). Start on the outside and work up to the top and across to the inside.
2. Holding the top of the toe with the left hand, thumb across the bottom of the toe (neck) in three rows starting from the bottom. Keeping your thumb at the back of the toe, use the index finger to caterpillar across the front of the toe (throat) three rows.
3. Holding the foot with the left hand, use your right thumb to work up inside the second toe until you get to the top and then start at the bottom of the outside of the toe and work up. Make little circular rotations at the padded part of the top of the toe and give it a gentle tug (sinuses). Repeat for the other toes. You may swap hands if it is more comfortable.

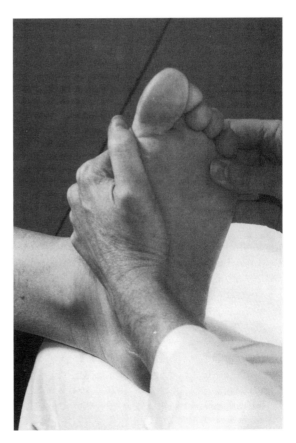

Working the lung area.

117

4. Thumb along the top of the ball of the foot with the right hand from inside out. Then supporting the foot with your right hand thumb back in the opposite direction with your left hand. Work along the ball of the foot in three rows from top to bottom (lungs).

5. Hold the foot with your right hand while you thumb downwards with your left hand from the little toe about an inch. Repeat this several times as this is an area that holds a lot of tension (shoulder).

6. Using fingers on both hands, massage in a circular motion around the ankle (adrenals and reproductive areas)

7. Take the foot and thumb downwards from the first joint of the big toe along the instep until you feel a protruding bone (navicular). Thumb across to the top of the the heel. Circle around the inside of heel. This represents the spine and thus links with the entire nervous system.

Repeat this sequence on the right foot.

Closing Sequence

1. Put your right fist into the ball of the right foot supporting with the left hand on the top side of the foot. Make a rotation with the fist and scoop up the instep.

2. Make a wringing action with your hands on the inside of the foot over the spine area.

3. Hold the feet together, side-by-side, and put your thumbs into each of the solar plexus areas. Get your partner to breathe in as you apply pressure with the thumbs and the feet flex up towards them. As they breathe out, release your thumbs and stretch their feet back towards you. Repeat a few times synchronizing your own breathing with the movement.

The pacing of your technique can either be slow, to encourage relaxation, or vigorous, to encourage stimulation. After the treatment, your partner should be encouraged to drink water. Sometimes they can feel a little headachy – this is caused by the release of toxins in the body. Just rest and drink lots of water. Often a treatment can make someone feel a bit sleepy so it should not be done just before a performance. Your feet should feel like new and with this increased awareness you can now approach the exercises.

Grounding Work

The following exercises help you to pay attention to what is going on in the feet. This restored body intelligence gives you many important clues as to what is occurring elsewhere in the body. Often, imbalances that occur in the pelvis and head actually manifest themselves in our walking habits. An awareness of this can be the first step in realigning ourselves. Take a look at an old pair of shoes and see how the undersides have been worn down. You may notice considerable differences between the two shoes in terms of which parts of the soles and heels have taken the pressure. We can begin to read our shoes to give us valuable information about the way we use our bodies. An awareness of this is very helpful in bodywork and builds up a whole picture of our body use that we can then relate to episodes in our lives. The foot can be a meaningful place to begin an autobiographical exploration of our past. Potentially, both the psychological and physical information that comes out of this enquiry can be tremendously revealing for us in our creative work. As the eminent reflexologist Laura Norman tells us, 'We walk on our soles/souls.'

Base Triangle

Keeping your feet firmly placed on the ground, spend some time shifting the weight through different areas of the feet. See what happens to the weight distribution throughout the body as you reorganize yourself around the different points of contact. Return to what feels like an even distribution and notice whether you naturally give more weight to one foot than the other and whether your weight is more on one side of the feet than the other. What is going on with the ankles? Is one side dropped? Do you tend to push into the front of your foot or towards the back? Ideally, you should think of an even balance of the triangle made by the base of the big toe, the base of the little toe and the heel.

Shifting Sands

Here is an Alexander-type exercise that requires a lot of concentration but that really helps you connect with the feet and indeed the whole of your lower body. As you are performing the exercise, be careful to keep your neck soft with the spine long and free as the effort of focusing the attention through the lower body can sometimes cause the shoulders, back and neck to tighten up.

1. Stand with feet in parallel, hip-width apart, with a feeling of length in the spine. You should have a sensation that your head is just lightly balanced on your neck. If you had a mirror in front of you, you would notice if your head were tilting slightly to one side or tipping either forward or back. Have a sense of total evenness so that if you were bisected down the front, each half would be symmetrical. Make any adjustment.
2. Close your eyes and put your attention into your pelvis, legs and feet. Check that your weight is evenly distributed. Keep breathing well and be aware of being soft and free in your neck. Let your shoulders be loose and allow the spine to lengthen. Breathe through the soles of your feet.
3. Now, close your eyes and imagine that your right leg is filled with grains of sand, a bit like the sand shifting through an egg-timer. Slowly feel the weight of the sand taking your body weight over towards that side. The left leg will feel light and comparatively empty.
4. Now, imagine that the grains of sand are shifting very slowly, grain by grain up through the top of the thigh into the pelvis and down to begin to fill the left leg. Slowly, the right leg empties and the left leg begins to bear weight. Feel it filling up all the way from the foot to the top of the thigh. There will come a point when the left leg feels much more weighted and your body will shift naturally over to this side.
5. Slowly begin to return the sand back through the pelvis. When the two halves of the body have equal weight, open your eyes and breathe freely. Repeat several times and feel what has

happened to the sensation of your body. If you have done the exercise mindfully and without rushing, you should now be feeling more grounded.

Tiptoe to Squat Balance – Working from the Air to the Earth

This exercise is particularly strengthening for the arch of the foot that in many people has a tendency to fall. As we have seen in reflexology, this area is strongly connected with the spine. People with flat feet often have back problems because they are lacking a stable triangular base and collapse inward.

1. Stand with the feet hip-width apart, arms hanging loosely by the side. Focus your attention on the contact you are making with the feet on the ground. Have a sensation of breathing through the soles of the feet.
2. Keep the neck soft and free and let the arms just drop loosely to the side. Breathe in and keeping a sense of length on the spine, rise up onto tiptoes, and hold for a few breaths. Now, still on tiptoes, lower yourself slowly into a squat, trying to keep your balance. Use your arms to help you. Feel the sacrum dropping to the ground to lengthen your lower back.
3. Stay on the balls of your feet keeping the spine long.
4. Hold for a few long breaths, then rise up to standing, still on the balls of your feet, then lower the heels to the ground. Take two breaths and repeat the exercise through rising to squatting and standing three times.

Salute to the Earth

This grounding yoga sequence is adapted from a variety of classic asanas and works with gravity to connect you powerfully to the earth energy. It also helps to strengthen the hip area and is often recommended for pregnant women. Many problems in the feet originate from tight lower backs and hip flexors and this sequence is particularly remedial. Try repeating *Salute to the Earth* three times and note how the sensations of being grounded gradually intensify. Use mats to protect your knees.

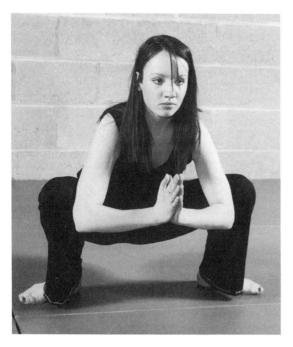

Earth squat.

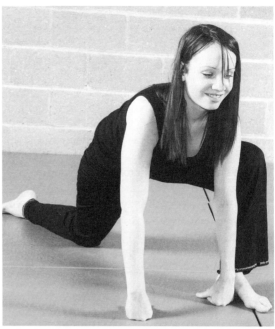

Earth rocking lunge.

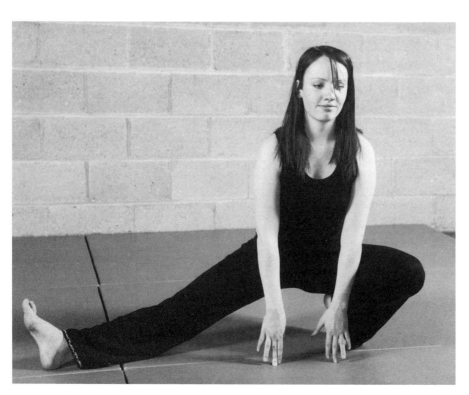

Earth squat with leg extended.

1. Stand with the feet parallel and with the palms together in prayer position. Breathe in.
2. Turning the toes out, take your feet hip-width apart and on the exhalation, slowly lower your body into a squat. If you can, keep the heels down and press them into the ground. If it's difficult to balance, stay up on the balls of your feet and try not to tip forward.
3. With hands still in prayer position, press the elbows against the inner thighs to encourage the knees and hips to open. Keeping the spine long, breathe three times.
4. Come up onto the ball of your left foot and extend your right leg out to the side of your body. Flex the right foot and balance with your fingertips in front of you trying to maintain the length of the spine. Take three long breaths.
5. Now, bring your right leg in and kneeling up onto this knee, bend your left knee up and step onto this foot. Place your hands on the floor inside your left foot and rock forward and back through a rocking lunge action, breathing out as you move forward and in as you move backwards. Repeat three times.
6. Bring your right leg in and kneel on both knees. Centre yourself in the kneeling position with your hands in prayer and take three long breaths.
7. Now still kneeling, and keeping your bottom as low as possible, open your knees and lower your trunk between your legs, keeping the spine as long as possible. Breathe three times, resting in this central earthing position. Stay longer if you want to – this is a very restorative place to be.

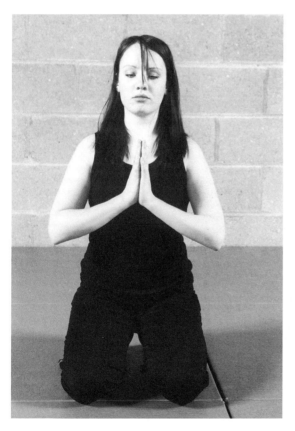

Earth kneeling prayer.

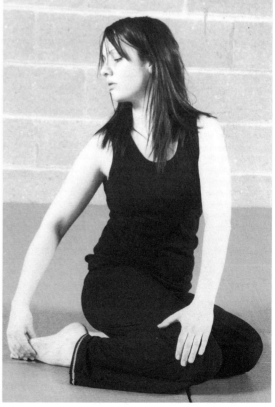

Earth sitting twist.

8. Raise trunk and, bringing your knees together, place your bottom on the floor to the left of your feet. Now, rotate your body in a twisting action to the right and look over your right shoulder. The spine should be long and lifted and the neck soft. Allow the shoulders to slide down the back. The left hand should be on your right knee and the right hand should be on your right foot, using your thumb to press into the ball of the foot. This is a revitalizing shiatsu point (KD 1).

9. Return through the centre and now repeat from 8 on the opposite side.
10. You now repeat all the movements through the opposite side of the body in reverse order before returning yourself finally to standing.

The cyclical nature of this sequence itself feels very grounding. Having performed it a few times, you will feel the calming effects of the earth energy and experience a lowering of your centre of

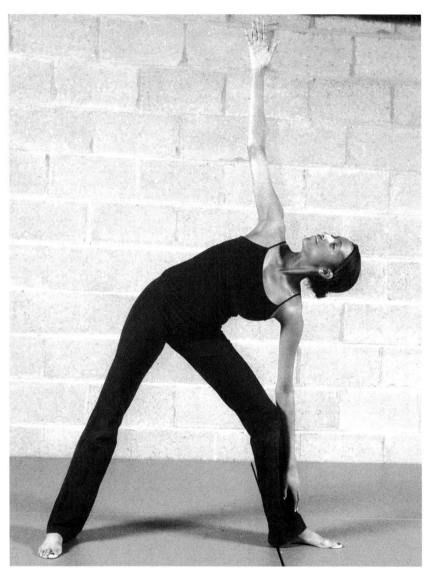

Triangle pose.

gravity. Performing this sequence can have a lowering effect on the voice, making it deeper and richer. *Salute to the Earth* contrasts with the fire energy experienced in *Salute to the Sun*, conferring a sense of security and stability to both mind and body. *Salute to the Earth* can be particularly useful when having to play very physical characters to get a strong sense of the grounded body and voice.

Triangle Pose

This is one of the classic yoga standing asanas, bringing stamina and strength. Its power depends on the contact of the back leg into the ground. It is this grounding action that allows the spine to lengthen and extend away. Use a non-slip yoga mat.

1. Stand tall with feet together. Breathe in and on the exhalation, jump the feet about a metre apart, into a parallel position. Turn the right foot out 90 degrees and turn the left foot slightly in.
2. Breathe in and on an exhalation, incline the trunk towards the right side with a sense that the base of the spine is releasing towards the left to allow the spine to elongate towards the head. The feeling should be that with each exhalation the navel moves back towards the spine, allowing the waist to lengthen and soften. Continue to breathe, playing with this sensation.
3. Allow the back foot to press firmly into the ground as the leg lengthens away. This provides a strong resistance for the spine to lengthen in the opposite direction.
4. In the early stages, you don't have to straighten the right leg or you may lock into the pose. However, do make sure that the right knee is not straying beyond the right ankle as this could cause injury.
5. When you have tuned into the release occurring in the spine, take the right hand down towards the right leg and allow the left arm to float up into the air. Don't be in a hurry to fix the arms in position but instead feel the lengthening in the spine first, and only when

you are ready, let the arms release out and away from the body's centre. The feeling is that the arms extend like wings, from the central core of the body.
6. Keep playing with the sensation of the foot rooted into the ground and the spine growing away. If you get tired, come up and rest and then move into the position once more.
7. Now try the triangle pose on the other side.

Warrior Pose

The very title gives a strong indication of the nature of this pose forming a useful preparation for a sense of impetus and steadfastness in performance. The warrior pose is a classic standing asana gathering its power from the feet. The orthodox way of doing this pose is with both feet flat on the floor. Another effective way of experiencing it is to balance the back foot on the *ball* of the foot and push away from that point. This almost gives the sensation of a sprung foot or of working from a starting block.

1. Start with feet together in parallel and take a long stride forward, bending the front leg so that the thigh is at 90 degrees to the calf.
2. Press down onto the ball of the back foot and feel the connection of this action to the spine that lifts up in response to this resistance. Feel the base of the spine sinking downwards and the waist lengthening. Hips should be in line so that the body is centred.
3. Hands can be in prayer position or alternatively, the arms lengthen upwards away from the body, without strain. Breathe clearly, drawing back the navel on each exhalation.

Exercises to Help You Develop Playfulness
Tennis Ball Massage

This exercise is useful for those who feel uncomfortable with having their feet touched and can be used for individual and ensemble activities. Place a tennis ball on the floor and roll this under the sole of your right foot. Really root the left foot in the ground to give you connection to the earth and to stabilize yourself. Make sure that knees are soft at all times. Experiment with rolling the ball under

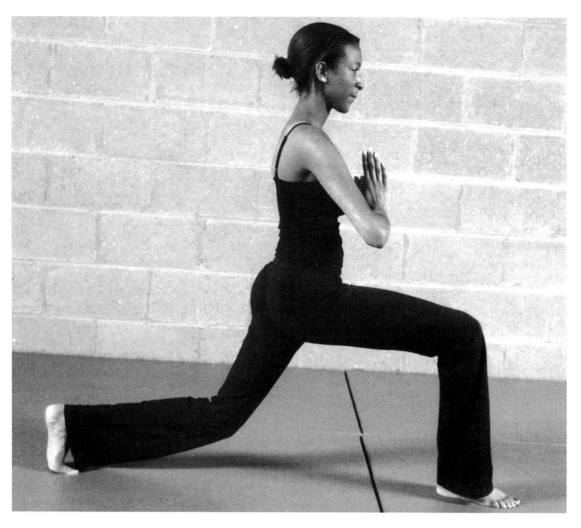

Warrior pose.

the sole of the foot and see what sensations this arouses. Remember to work the arch of the foot as it connects with the spinal area.

Standing, Water Visualization
Stand, breathing through the soles of the feet. It is a really hot day. Your feet are sore, swollen and tired. Scrunch your toes up under you to give you a tight, bound sensation. Then opening out your toes and letting the whole surface of the foot make contact with the ground, imagine you are standing now on cool, soft grass. Take a few steps towards an

imaginary stream. Step in slowly. Feel the coolness lapping up to your ankles. Walk through the icy cold stream of water, sensing the coolness travelling up your legs and into your body, making you feel refreshed. You are aware of small currents of water lapping over your feet. Notice how your walk feels sensual as your legs feel connected into your hips. Observe how your breath connects you to the feet. Picking up one foot, choose someone else in the room and splash them with water by kicking your foot through the water and towards your target! Receive their splash on your own body and begin a water fight exchange solely through the feet.

Walking Meditation

After using the imagination in the previous exercise, this is a good way of getting some physical experience of the sensuality of the foot. It is common practice in Buddhist meditation to walk barefoot on a variety of surfaces. Even in freezing conditions, the experience of connecting with the ground through bare feet is invigorating. Walking is done at a slow, even pace with a sense of a backward wheel motion. Be mindful of the way the surface of the foot makes contact with the ground and rolls from the heel through the ball to the toes. Keep the hands folded over the dan tien and look straight ahead. Experiment with walking over a variety of surfaces preferably outdoors. The even rhythm of your breathing should correspond with your walking pace. Bring your attention to the relationship between the breath and the texture underfoot.

Picking up Objects with Feet

Gather together an interesting collection of objects ranging from feathers to keys to small pieces of jewellery and fabrics such as old silk scarves. See how easy each item is to pick up. See if you can pass objects to a partner, using only the soles of your feet. If you can build up dexterity in this area, try then to work with chalks and paper to create art work.

Feldenkrais Footwork from the Floor

Revisit the foot-led Feldenkrais work explored in Chapter 2 before experimenting with the following exercise.

Foot to Foot Contact Work

This next exercise is performed with a partner. Ambient music would be helpful.

1. Lie foot to foot with your partner on a couple of mats that will support and protect both your entire lengths. Get close enough together so that the soles of your feet are touching but your legs are not quite straight. You should feel comfortably connected to your partner without feeling that they are on top of you. Spend some time now just 'listening' to your partner's feet. See if you can tune into the feet as live and sentient parts of their being.

2. Allow yourself to begin to move first one pair of soles and then the other. You will naturally want to investigate the space above the mat after a while rather than staying rooted to ground level. See whether the feet want to move in the same or a counterpointed rhythm. Who is leading the movement, your foot or your partner's? Is there a way you can alternate the initiative. It may be that you exchange the impulse to lead or it may be that for some time, one foot or pair of feet is far more energetic.

3. As you begin to be more adventurous you will find that the hips and lower body will shift as part of the natural rhythm of the movement originating from the foot. Go with this and see what happens. Eventually, this will become a foot duet. Don't force or pre-think the movements: it works best if you can respond to an instinctive sense of where to go next. Give your foot its head and leave your brain out of it. If in doubt or if you lose the connection, keep breathing through your feet and maintain contact with your partner's energy.

4. This exercise can go on for around fifteen minutes and still be transforming and developing. Eventually let your feet slowly come apart and rest in semi-supine tuning into your body and your breath, noticing any alteration in your state of being. It is natural to feel a slight sense of disconnection and loss once you separate from your footmate.

Creative Work with Shoes

Working with shoes can provide a powerful stimulus to creativity. Many physical theatre companies, such as Told by an Idiot, have used shoes as a catalyst into improvisation. Worn shoes have a very personal character and these can provoke some highly charged emotional responses. As a preparation to this work get a sense of your own shoe's history and those of the group.

1. Stand in a circle with your shoes off and just one of them by your side. Someone throws one of their shoes to someone who sends it to another until it has been passed around the whole group.
2. Keep the sequence of throwing in the same order and add another shoe, so that two shoes are being thrown at the same time. Don't worry about dropping the shoe – just retrieve it and carry on throwing to your partner.
3. See if you can introduce all the shoes. This requires extreme concentration as you have to throw whilst looking back to catch at the same time. Each of the shoes will have different weights, textures and smells, deeply linked to individual members of the group.

The following exercise requires some atmospheric music to stimulate a creative background context.

1. Gather together a pile of old shoes from wardrobe stock or a charity shop.
2. Each person chooses a shoe that they feel speaks to them.
3. Spend some time examining your shoe, feeling its weight in your hands, smelling its character, observing where it is worn, even trying it on if this feels appropriate.
4. Slowly begin to move with the shoe, not necessarily just wearing it, allowing a sense of the shoe's owner and your relationship to them to emerge. Your movement will be affected by your 'memory' of this imagined person, and

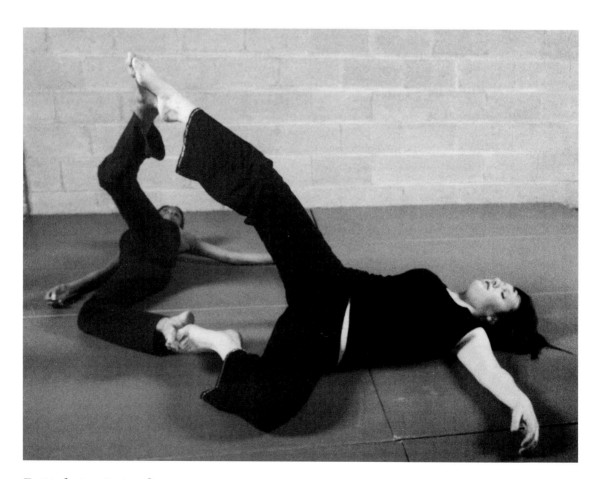

Foot to foot contact work.

might express any one of a variety of moods; nostalgic, mournful, celebratory, fearful, or contradictory.
5. Allow the music to inform your responses as an imagined history begins to emerge.

This exercise might be usefully undertaken in relation to a character within a production that you are working on.

Mythologies of the Foot

In fairy stories throughout Europe it is surprising how often the foot comes up as a signifier. Primitive emotions are expressed through the feet – remember *Rumplestiltskin* stamping his feet in anger? The foot is a metaphor for powerful, often violent feelings and for the passionate expression of repressed emotions. You may also know the story of *The Twelve Dancing Princesses* who wore out their shoes going to a secret kingdom and dancing ecstatically all night long until morning. And Cinderella's little foot was an object of desire when she lost a glass slipper and gained a prince. Contained in these stories are important gender notions surrounding identity and images of femininity and desire. Perhaps the most interesting fairy story concerning feet is *The Red Shoes* where the heroine's passionate and compulsive dancing releases unbridled feelings. These primitive forces are viewed by society as dangerous and consequently prohibited. The conflict is between domesticity and sobriety, represented by sensible shoes, and self-expression represented by the dancing red shoes. In Freudian psychoanalysis the foot is connected to the *id* (primitive self) as opposed to the head that houses the *ego*. Primitive expression is often sexual and the foot has been fetishized with heels, buckles and bows. The sexualized form of expression can be a source of creative energy.

The Red Shoes – Synopsis of Story

Most people are familiar with the part of the story in which the heroine, intoxicated with dance, is unable to remove the red shoes and dances herself into a frenzy. Less well known, is that at the beginning of the story, the girl has a highly playful and natural connection with her feet, and fashions herself a pair of 'home-made' shoes from red felt. Later, in the house of the old woman, her adoptive mother, she is made to give these up and wear a pair of sensible black shoes. This results in a symbolic closing down of her creative spirit. She becomes frustrated and rebellious and resorts to deceit when she substitutes the black for red shoes that she dares to wear in church. She continues to play with fire, taking more and more risks as she dances herself into a delirious state. Eventually, tormented by the shoes that she cannot take off, she begs a woodcutter to chop them off.

It is possible to think about the story in terms of a series of metaphors. Feminist psychologist Clarissa Pinkola Estes has analyzed this story and identified the heroine's passage through four distinct states of being, from innocence through to bitter experience. We might usefully relate these phases to Gabrielle Roth's *Five Rhythm Movement* theory, outlined below.

Gabrielle Roth's Five Rhythms

The *Five Rhythms* form part of a theory of movement developed by the inspirational American dancer, Gabrielle Roth, in which Five distinctive Rhythms – flow, staccato, chaos, lyrical and stillness – are identified as being common to all cultures and potentially present within each individual. Each of the Rhythms has a particular psychological as well as physical resonance. *Five Rhythms* workshops involve the participants moving to carefully selected music and discovering their personal responses to the Rhythms on a deep somatic level.

The experience of working with the Rhythms can be personally illuminating, depending on which rhythm one feels most at ease with and if any feel difficult or alien. Some people, for example, find staccato a challenging place to be since it is a combative, assertive, even fierce Rhythm and, depending on our upbringing, we may feel uneasy about being in this rhythmic place. The fourth Rhythm, chaos, is one that many people find especially tough to connect with. This is because, as the name implies, chaos involves a state of completely letting go and being unreservedly expressive in response to the impulses of the music. The reason it may be so hard to respond to is that we are rarely encouraged to abandon ourselves in such a primal and uninhibited way, beyond pre-conceived levels of respectability. Truly responding to the chaos rhythm requires a total surrender to disorientation as our subconscious responses kick in and the rational mind is left floundering. A superficial response to chaos is often easily achieved, by simulating a club-like atmosphere, but a genuine experience of this rhythm goes much deeper.

Within each of her designated Five Rhythms, Roth defines further archetypal qualities so that at an advanced level, one can discover resonances with some potentially highly sophisticated move-ment states through this work. Even at their simplest level though, the *Five Rhythms* offer powerfully contrasting experiential states, a brief summary of which is given below:

- Flow – a 'feminine' rhythm, sensual, curving, fluent, confident, earthy, free-flowing, fecund, deep; a child playing knowing exactly what to do next
- Staccato – a 'masculine' rhythm, jagged, energetic, sharply defined, explosive, dynamic, electric, potentially dangerous. At its best, it generates order, discipline and leadership, if misused it can generate a feeling of empty conformity, even sterility
- Chaos – wilderness, a no-man's land beyond the pale. A therapeutic place to be for a short while, providing one can get back from this rhythm by careful earthing
- Lyrical – a 'poetic' space, lyrical often leads us 'upwards' towards a spiritual place, enjoying a feeling of lightness, dreaminess and trans-parency
- Stillness – not just emptiness, but a feeling of charged reflection, a gathering of all the other experience from a place of calm. Think of the movement of spinning and then stopping and the dynamism within that moment of stillness.

The Red Shoes will give you a feel for Five Rhythms work in response to a story that incorporates some of these movement states. Indicated in the text are

areas where a practical experience of the Five Rhythms would be enriching.

The Red Shoes – a Movement Workshop

As a preliminary, perform the reflexology sequence and some grounding exercises given above. This will sensitize you and prepare you to relate creatively to the various phases of the story that are outlined below, and carefully chosen music for each state.

You will require some strips of red material, a red high-heeled shoe, a large bowl of water and a towel.

For the state of childish innocence and invention (Lyrical and Flow), perform some of the *playfulness* exercises described earlier to experience some of the rhythms of flow and lyrical. The following movement exercise will help you connect to the playful state. Prepare some strips of red fabric cut up from lengths of material. Reread the part of the story where the girl makes her hand-made red shoes. This is a time in her life of self-sufficiency and pleasurable inventiveness. It relates to a time when she could play all day and be endlessly resourceful.

1. Gently wrap each foot in red strip red cloth. Lie on your back in semi-supine and gently wriggle your feet. Enjoy the sensation of movement in your feet. Hold your toes and improvise bending and stretching your legs alternately. Don't be afraid to roll and shift your weight on your back. Experiment with the patterns your feet can make in the air.
2. Roll over onto all fours and from here roll up to standing. Work with some powerful rhythmic music and allow yourself to travel and skip experimenting with all the different rhythms your feet can make. Your movements are very free but still controlled and gentle. All the movements come from the floor upward and are accompanied by a feeling of delight and playfulness.
3. You should feel as though you are listening to your feet to which you are very attached. This should feel a very natural and harmonious state of being, in which you are free to be

spontaneous and yet remain in control. There should be a sense of pleasure and satisfaction in your movements as you follow your impulses and yet feel quite secure. Quite often, by the time we reach adulthood, we become pre-occupied with following rules; as a result we lose connection with this freely inventive state of being and, consequently, our ability to improvise playfully is affected.

The Repressed State (Staccato)

This relates to the section of the story in which the girl is forced into black 'sensible' shoes and enters a state of joylessness and repression. We can all remember a period in our lives when we have to give up our spontaneity and lead a more regulated and uniform life that may involve walking in step with others and sublimating impulsive behaviour.

1. So, take off your hand-made red shoes and put them away out of sight. As you do this, have a sense of the symbolic meaning of this sur-rendering of playfulness and loss of your inventive self.
2. Standing, feel tension in your whole body, beginning with the feet. Have a sense that the freedom of movement has seized up as you begin to move mechanically in hard, angular lines. Experiment with a staccato type move-ment that might involve marching, slashing or other repetitive actions. Move in slow motion as you repeat these actions so you simulate a sense of monotony and dreariness. Your move-ments should feel dull and uninspired. Have a feeling that you are losing motivation and energy and have to drag yourself through the repeated actions. The keynote here is con-formity and a lack of zest.

The Manic State (Chaos)

The reaction against the repressed state is a desire to kick out. Like all rebellions, this can sometimes be a violent experience. Remember, in the story, the frenzied dancing culminates in her 'losing her head' and being unable to control herself. This is an exhilarating but also very dangerous state to be in as it can lead to addictions (promiscuity,

drug-taking, self-harming, eating disorders). The following exercises will help you connect with the heightened energy and risk-taking. It's helpful to get a primal rhythm going by beginning with some music that you find compulsive to dance to. Now try some of the following.

1. Spinning as fast and as long as you can.
2. Jumps from standing – leaping into the air with a sense of gleeful defiance.
3. Exploring forbidden space. Over the head, or behind you – using your body in an unexpected and startling way.
4. Everybody runs around the space, changing direction constantly. One person picks up a red high-heeled shoe and with a sense of its symbolic sensuality throws it from person to person. Once caught, the receiver rolls on the floor and then flings it to the next person. The rhythm should be fast and furious.
5. Dancing on imaginary hot coals, pushing through the pain barrier, allow this to develop into chaotic movement that's both seductive and potentially damaging.

The Recovery State (Stillness)

1. After passing through the fire of the manic state in the original *Red Shoes*, the central character finds relief through the brutal act of the feet being chopped off. Here we may recover the more innocent state by simply lying down and allowing the breath to calm the body. Regain a connection with the security of the ground and experience the calm after the storm.
2. When you feel restored, sit up and gently stroke the feet to soothe. Stand up and plunge your feet in the bowl of water. This ritual act of cleansing will help to heal the rebellious foot and restore a sense of wholeness so that the foot reconnects with the rest of the body. Remember what the imaginary water felt like in the visualization exercise in Chapter 6 and try to recover that sense of innocence.
3. Wipe the feet dry and then go and take out the red strips of fabric. Put these back onto the feet, and as you do so have a sense of all you have

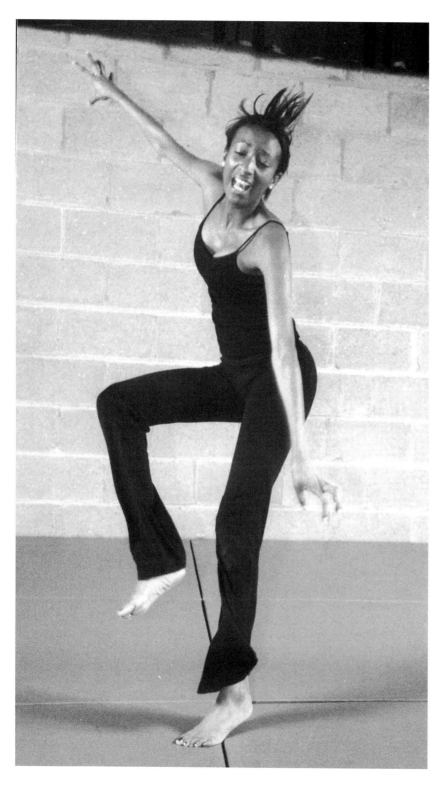

The Red Shoes – *chaos state.*

passed through. Start to re-explore the feet in the space with a sense of wisdom and reflection. Tranquil music may be helpful to produce an atmosphere of the return to 'home', after a long and challenging journey.

The journey of the feet in these exercises takes us through rites of passage on a quest for the self. Experiencing the rhythms is part of such a journey into self-awareness. It is only through knowing ourselves that we can truly ground ourselves. The more grounded we are, the higher we can jump.

There is a Zen saying: 'The wise man breathes through his feet not through his throat', and indeed it is extraordinary how having a renewed sense of our feet on the ground improves the quality of both respiration and voice. The final chapter turns our attention to breath. It is by tapping into the body's potential through the breath that the performer is released into a journey of self-awareness and creativity.

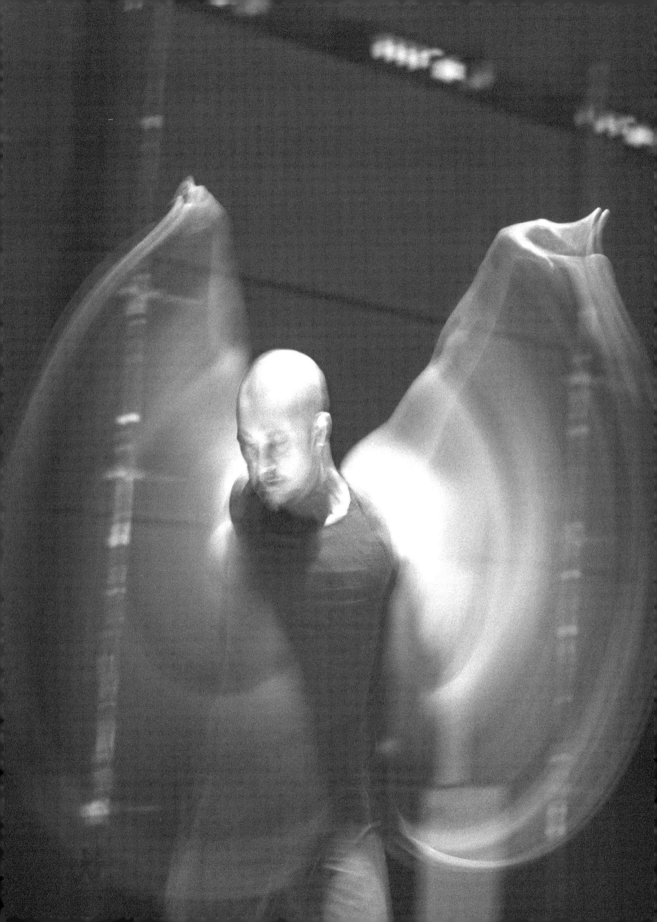

7 THE BREATH

Many of the practices we have been exploring in the previous chapters centre themselves in the experience of breathing and indeed the attention to breath is one of the defining qualities of holistic bodywork. This chapter draws together some of these practices through a focus on the crucial role of breathing in connecting the physical and the metaphysical.

In everyday life we rarely give our breath a second thought. Nor do we need to, since it's a function of the autonomic nervous system. Because of this, we often take our breath for granted, failing to use it to the full except in situations where extraordinary demands are placed on the body. Pregnant women are taught to use their breath to manage the pain of labour and to help to facilitate effective muscle use in giving birth, yet rarely do we engage in any development of our breathing to help cope with the pressures of ordinary life. Indeed, we only become aware of our breathing at all during times of intense emotion, for example, when we are scared or trying to control our anger.

Breathing is intimately bound up with our emotion, hence the changes to our breath when we laugh or cry or dream. Being able to recognize our emotions and stay in touch with them through breathing practices is a valuable skill for the expressive performer. The great experimental French director Antonin Artaud, believed that different parts of our body related to different emotions, and these could be reached and retrieved on what he called the 'whetted edge of his breathing'. Such an idea no longer seems outlandish when we begin to appreciate the intimate relationship between mind and body. Our breath represents the living interface of that relationship and provides a valuable means of sourcing body memory.

Breathing and Performance

Of course, the way we breathe is reflected in the way we stand, move and speak, either freely and lightly, or tightly and withheld. It is useful to first engage with this awareness in our own bodies, since so often performance work requires us to observe the effect of the internal rhythm of breath on the characters/moods we are trying to bring to life. One of the key areas we might explore when creating a character or state of being is the breathing. Is it fast, slow, sluggish, excitable, sensuous, timid? Addressing the breath will take us right into the centre of the character's psycho-physicality. Yet only when we understand and have some control over our own breathing patterns can we begin to infuse life into our characterizations through breath.

Breathing has both a physiological and a psychological aspect and the two are related. We have already noted how in performance fear and self-consciousness can undermine the breath and hence our capacity for expression. By cultivating good breathing, we can combat this danger and regain purpose and confidence. We know how in martial arts the appropriate mustering of breath helps the warrior towards a lethal delivery. In the same way, the performer can draw on a powerful sense of focus by connecting both physical and mental resources on and through the breath.

Fundamentally, it is our breathing that determines the quality of our energy and wellbeing. To breathe is our most primordial instinct. Our life-force depends on the act of breathing as we use the oxygen to convert our food into sensation, movement, feeling and thought and to aid in the process

OPPOSITE: Akram Khan in Kaash.
Photograph by Roy Peters

133

of cell renewal and growth. If we don't breathe properly, we become listless and don't operate at our full capacity. Moreover, poor breathing affects our ability to speak, move and concentrate: all of which are essential qualities for a performer.

In this final chapter we will be dealing with four interrelated routes to the breath and breathing:

- the physiology of breathing;
- breathing with energy and movement;
- breathing and voice;
- breathing and meditation.

Benefits of Cultivating the Breath

The Cultivation of Effective Breathing Helps the Performer

- It supports good body use, essential to unforced performance.
- Helps to keep the mind focused and tranquil, ready to respond to the challenges of rehearsal and performance.
- Supports the unrestricted flow of voice and sound, phrase and movement.
- Releases a powerful source of energy and maintains a healthy yin/yang balance.
- Wards off the detrimental effects of tension, stress and stage fright.
- Allows effective use of bodywork practices, beneficial to creative work.
- Improves grace, flow and centering in the whole being.
- Allows us to ground our work and control our responses both within and without.
- Helps us to understand and manifest the links between breath and expression.

The Physiology of Breath

Don't Force the Breath

In trying to increase the breath we often artificially lengthen our breathing by an act of sheer will. We will never get anywhere by clenching the teeth and commanding the breath. The breath has to be gently coaxed. One way of getting around this trap

of struggling for a deeper breath is to calmly observe oneself breathing, rather than fretfully forcing a deeper breath. Think of yourself as split in two – a breathing self and a witness. This allows a sense of detachment.

When you first practise breathing with awareness you may prefer to lie down to observe the rise and fall of the belly as the diaphragm expands and contracts and to feel for this movement by placing your fingertips lightly on your abdomen. Supine is the best way to monitor the breath without imposing a sense of strain on the body. This position discourages the shoulders from tensing and getting caught up in the breathing action. As you are breathing, remind yourself that the lungs don't just exist at the front of the body but go right through to the back of the body near to the spine and back ribs. Having this sense of the lungs being behind as well as in the front of the body, helps us to increase the volume of the breath by expanding the back ribs and allowing the lungs to rush into this additional space. This visualization of the back of the body during breath also helps to re-energize the spine and after a while, you may even be able to feel an increased sensation on the spine as the lungs fill into this area to take in oxygen.

The Cycle of Inhalation and Exhalation

The more air we can exhale, and the more relaxed our breathing apparatus, the better the quality of the inhalation bringing new oxygen to the lungs, blood and cells of the body. When you hold your breath, you store up carbon dioxide and this builds up in the muscles and can be weakening. It is impossible to exhale all the stale air from the lungs. Like a dirty teacup, there will always be a few dregs left at the bottom. However, there are various ways of encouraging an improved draught of freshly inhaled air.

1. Allow a pause between inhalation and exhalation. Think of the air being exhaled, like a bucket being passed down a well. Try and count the exhalation down the well, on a count of eight. At the bottom of the well, the bucket pauses to take up a fresh bucketful on the inbreath. During this pause, wait on the count of

four before drawing up the new bucket of freshly oxygenated air over a count of eight. Because of the wait, the lungs are eager and ready to draw breath and the breath will be deeper and longer than if you had not paused. At the top of the inhalation, pause again for four before resuming the cycle. As the breathing settles try to increase the length of time you are counting.

2. Another way to improve the quality of the breath is to exhale normally and then, on a sharply aspirated sound, push the residue of air out of the lungs. Think of the dregs in the teacup and expel them over the edge. The next in breath will be longer and thirstier for the emptying action of the previous exhalation.

A Sharp Intake of Breath
When we need to take in a maximum amount of oxygen in a short space of time we breathe through the mouth. The slower and more relaxed way of breathing is to inhale through the nose and out through the mouth. This enables the jaw to soften so that the airways are relaxed. In general, we tend to exhale on the point of effort, whether that be physical or vocal. As a result, many performers need to develop the extended exhalation in order to carry a phrase, movement or note. You can redo the previous exercise extending the out breath.

Note: Remember that deep breathing exercises can result in dizziness and hyperventilation if not done with caution. Make sure there is fresh air and take a short walk around the room in between exercises. If, during these exercises you begin to feel dizzy, stop immediately, sit down and put your head between your legs. Should you feel you are going to hyperventilate, cross your arms over your chest to reduce the intake of oxygen and concentrate on breathing out for as long as you can.

Two Types of Breathing
Fundamentally, it is helpful to divide breathing into two separate physiological processes.

- *From the outside in* – the mechanical action of drawing oxygen from the outside into the respiratory system, and expelling carbon dioxide through the same route once the air has been used in the body.
- *Cellular breathing* – the chemical exchange of gases that takes place in the cells of the body as oxygen enters and carbon dioxide is expelled.

Being conscious of these processes can help us to improve the quality of our breathing.

From the Outside In
The first level of breathing involves the intake of air through the action of the diaphragm, a large muscle in the lower abdomen that sucks down and creates a vacuum in the lungs. Air is drawn in through the nose and so into the trachea (windpipe) and then on into the bronchi, and lungs. Once in the lungs, the breath passes into the alveoli, tiny air-sacs, resembling clusters of myriad, grape-like structures. If opened out and stretched flat the surface area of the alveoli would cover a football pitch, forty times larger than the surface area of the skin. The lungs are protected by ribs that connect in the front of the body to the breastbone and at the back of the body with the thoracic spinal vertebrae. When we breathe in, these ribs expand sideways to permit the expansion of the lungs. Two lower 'floating' ribs are only connected to the breastbone and are 'free' at the back to allow even greater expansion. Healthy breathing depends on the free movement of the ribs and the spine and many of the exercises explored in this chapter are designed to develop this movement of the bones involved in the action of breathing. We shouldn't really separate our understanding of breathing from the need for easy movement in these key physical regions. The Feldenkrais work explored earlier in the book is particularly helpful for releasing the bones and the muscles involved in breathing.

We start with the classic yoga exercise *Alternate Nostril Breathing* that focuses attention on the breath, alternately through one side of the body and then the other. Although the attention is superficially on the nostrils and the nasal passages, the ultimate effect of the sequence is to bring the awareness down into each lung. The sitting position from which the exercise is performed, ensures a long lifted spine that allows the space for good lung capacity. As Feldenkrais reminded us 'good breathing means good posture and vice versa'.

Yoga Breathing Exercise – Alternate Nostril Sequence

Sit comfortably in a crossed-leg position. If necessary, sit on a large book or supportive cushion so that the spine can remain lifted as you perform the breathing sequence.

1. With your right hand, place your index, middle and ring fingers in the middle of your forehead between your eyebrows (the area known as the third eye or brow centre). Place your thumb over your right nostril to block the airways. Slowly take in a breath through your left nostril to a count of eight.
2. Hold the breath in this position for a count of four and then block up the left nostril with your little finger releasing the thumb to exhale to a count of eight through your right nostril. Hold for a count of four.
3. Now, using the same counts, inhale through the right nostril, block it up with the thumb and then release the left nostril. Hold for four as before. Keep repeating the cycle, but be careful not to force the breath as you may hyperventilate.
4. The idea behind keeping the fingers on the third eye is to connect both sides of the body and maintain awareness of being both in the body but also witnessing from the outside. This dual perspective is both balancing and calming.

Cellular Breathing

The second level of breathing, known as 'cellular', refers to the exchange of gases that takes place within each individual cell of the body once the oxygen has entered the bloodstream via minute blood vessels around the air-sacs in the lungs. Once the oxygen has been used by the body in the processes of movement, bodily functions, growth and cell renewal, the waste carbon dioxide then passes back through the cell walls to be expelled to the outside air during exhalation.

Cellular Breathing Visualization

Rather than confining our concept of breathing to what is going on in the lungs, try instead to follow the journey of the breath imaginatively into the very cells of the body. Focus on a part of the body that feels tight, sore or unresponsive. Imagine as you take a breath in, that the bright scarlet blood is pumping into these stuck areas from the central part of the body where the lungs are to the periphery, recharging and carrying away the stale, dull air. It is remarkable how taking the attention into the 'dead' area can bring about a powerful reawakening and release. Just imagine the replenishment of oxygen that is taking place at cellular level. Quite often you will feel a warmth and improved sense of vitality as the mind traces the body's sense of regenerated energy.

The Breathing Spot – Releasing the Caught Breath

This next exercise explores the connection between the breath and the spine in a resting position. Very often our breath feels as though it is getting trapped somewhere below the ribs on the back of the body. This is frequently a troubled *breathing spot* in our lower backs where the muscles on either side of the spine may have been holding tension or causing a sway-back action. This is because the lower spine in this place suddenly has no ribs to brace it and so is inclined to collapse. This can bring about a shearing action in the spine causing the breath to feel stuck.

1. Kneel on a mat or blanket and gently flatten the torso over the knees in the yoga child position (*see* Chapter 3). Either rest your arms alongside your trunk on the mat or, if it feels more comfortable, stretch them over the head so that they are resting on the ground.
2. Make sure that you are not 'holding' anywhere. If your knees or ankles feel sore, place a towel or small blanket between calves and thighs or under the feet to relieve any pressure. Any position where the heart can rest beneath the spine is extremely restorative.

3. Let a partner observe the lie of the back and gently lay their hands around the lower ribs at the *breathing spot*. Breathe into the hands on the back, imagining a continuous flow of breath through the spine.

4. During this directed breathing, both partners can visualize an unbroken line along the spine, through the vertebrae from the tailbone to the crown. It is helpful to have a sense of the navel floating up to reach the spine on the exhalation. Let the visualization be of an uninterrupted stream of golden light.

5. Softly begin to increase the length of the breathing. With each exhalation, the resting partners should allow themselves to slide forward and open out the trunk further, allowing the torso to be heavier and more in contact with the thighs. Try and feel the breath on the spine on the inhalation. At any point where the breath feels caught or tight, consciously breathe into that area to release. It is likely that this is where the spine is less flexible and is restricting the movement of the breath.

The Diaphragm: the Body's Equator

The crucial muscle involved in the action of breath is the diaphragm, the great dome-like sheath that is attached to the lower ribs, the spine and the ziphoid process of the sternum, and effectively separates the abdomen and the chest. What happens in breathing is that as the diaphragm contracts, it pulls down towards the pelvis, enlarging the space in the chest. Air rushes in to fill the vacuum, expanding the lungs and bringing about the inhalation. As the diaphragm releases, it rises back up, expelling air and bringing about the exhalation.

As far back as 1937, Mabel Todd in her book *The Thinking Body*, described the diaphragm as 'the equator of the body, the dividing line of two great halves of being, the conscious and the unconscious'. Perhaps what she meant by this is that it is through the highly physical act of our breathing that we become aware of the non-physical interior world of feelings and emotions. The diaphragm literally 'divides' the body but also signifies the interface between the 'abstract' world of emotion and memory and the 'palpable' world of the body.

Diaphragm Work from the Cat Position

A breathing practice that really helps us get in contact with the action of the diaphragm is the yoga breathing in the cat position where you can really observe the effects of the inner breath in the body. As you inhale, expand the chest but don't inflate the belly. On exhalation, suck in the belly as you squeeze the air out of the abdomen. Think about sucking up the breath through the belly button so that the diaphragm slides up under the ribs.

Pilates Breathing

We might compare this kind of breathing to the breathing advocated by the Pilates method, which is so fundamental to the Pilates' approach to strengthening the core abdominal muscles. In Pilates you are encouraged to expand the lower ribs and the belly on the inhalation and then on the exhalation draw in the stomach muscles from the pubic bone towards the spine at the navel, as if zipping up a pair of trousers. This actively engages the pelvic floor muscles as the abdominal muscles are hollowed and scooped upwards. The focus here is very much on the lower abdomen from the pelvic floor to the diaphragm, strengthening the dan tien area. To develop a heightened sensation of the action of the diaphragm, try the following Pilates exercise.

Lateral Breathing – Scarf Exercise

This can either be done in kneeling or sitting position.

1. Take a scarf and place it around the diaphragm area towards the bottom of the ribcage. Hold each end of the scarf firmly as it crosses over the centre of your torso. Keep shoulders relaxed and elbows softly to the side of the body.

2. Take a deep breath into your back and the sides of the ribcage, feeling resistance from the scarf. If it gets too tight, loosen off the scarf a little.

3. On the out breath try to pull the scarf a little tighter to get rid of those last dregs of breath. It is important to draw up the stomach muscles

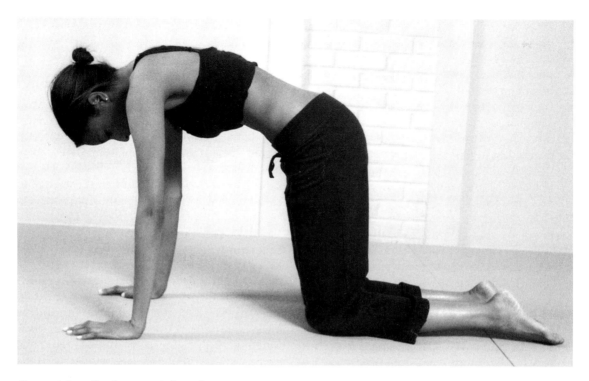

Cat position, diaphragmatic breathing.

from the pelvic floor towards the spine as you exhale. Repeat ten times.

This exercise should enable you to gain a greater awareness of the contribution of the lower back muscles to effective breathing. The aim is to strengthen the lower back, the abdominal muscles and the pelvic floor, that comprise the 'core'. A benefit of this kind of breathing is that it helps you to feel the connection between the two vertical layers of muscle comprising the pelvic floor and the diaphragm (relating in Ashtanga yoga to the lower and middle bandhas). Breathing tends to be nasal in both the Pilates and yogic practices.

Ujjayi Breathing and the Whispered 'Ah'
There is a specific yogic breathing technique called *ujjayi* or victorious breath, associated with Ashtanga that makes a sibilant sound through the throat. To find this, it is helpful to drop the chin, contracting the glottis at the back of the throat.

When you inhale and exhale deeply, again through the nose, a kind of soft snoring sound is made (like Darth Vader). The friction of air that makes the sibilant sound has the effect of warming and calming. This is particularly helpful for preparing the voice for performance. Practising ujjayi breathing with an awareness of the bandhas helps to release the energy associated with these important locations.

Advanced students of the Alexander Technique may be familiar with the 'whispered ah' that involves a comparable use of the breath.

1. In standing position (ensuring that the neck is free, head forward and up, and back wide and long), bend the knees and drop the pelvis, allowing the body to tip forward, keeping the spine long (monkey pose).
2. Now drop the jaw to an open-mouth position and place the tip of the tongue at the back of the lower teeth.

3. Thinking of something amusing (with a Mona Lisa smile) a sustained 'ah' sound is whispered through the mouth on the exhalation. Again this has the effect of preparing the voice for performance.

Breathing in Performance Training

It is not only the disciplines of yoga, Pilates and Alexander that have differing approaches to working with the breath. You may have experienced voice classes advocating yet further practices. A classic example is the instruction to expand the ribs high and wide while the diaphragm and abdominal muscles engage in contraction and expansion. The ribs are held in an expanded position whilst the diaphragm works to inhale and exhale. This rib expansion enables air to be stored in the rib cavity, retaining what is known as a 'rib-reserve' of breath. This is helpful in extending the breath to deal with long phrases or verse. The wind musician similarly develops breathing techniques to develop the breath, being supported from deep within the lower chest and back. The upper chest and shoulders become the last point of expansion on the in breath. This action helps to create the necessary power to support the resonance using the full bellows effect of the chest.

Whatever the method, all techniques draw attention to the importance of lower chest expansion and muscular control to develop the power of the diaphragm and the abdominal muscles in supporting the breath. As with any technique, the discipline of practice enables the breathing exercise to become habitual. Ultimately, it is important to find the technique that is comfortable for you and not get fixed in a mechanical approach that can distort the body and inhibit the free flow of breath.

On the Edge of Whetted Breath

Whatever technique you use in cultivating the breath, you will become increasingly aware of the exchange between the inhalation and exhalation. In this moment of dilation, the internal connects with the external, as your senses become heightened. It is a point of intense creativity akin to the Alexander Pause (moment of inhibition) and the split second when yin and yang energy transform. It is the pivotal space before exertion takes place and, in shiatsu terms, it is the instant when the practitioner enters into the body at a more profound level. Many contemporary practitioners since Artaud have appreciated this pregnant pause as potentially dynamic for the performer. Alternatively, the pause after the exhalation is a reflective moment that creates calm and deepens breathing. It is invaluable for the performer to develop an appreciation of these pivotal exchanges, and by doing some energy work with breath we can encourage a more active understanding.

Breath and Energy Channels and Movement

As seen in Chapter 4 breathing is used to enhance the flow of energy through the body, called *ki* or *prana*, which was traditionally used as a measure of a person's health and vitality. Breathing is significant not simply because it's the gateway to an elemental life force but because the taking in and expelling of air symbolizes the exchange that takes place between a person and the world outside. The quality of our breathing says something about how comfortable we are in our relationship with the world around us and how capable we are of making a full exchange. The most important thing is that, in an Alexander way, we don't interfere with our breathing by trying too hard or getting anxious, thus making the breathing shallow. Holistic practices can help to remedy these tendencies and give space for our breathing. Softer, fuller breathing then becomes habitual so that in times of acute stress or demands on the performer, the body remembers how to let go and replenish itself. The following exercise tunes us in to action of the yin gathering and yang expelling in a gentle and expansive way.

Tai Chi Lotus Breathing

1. Stand centred, knees slightly bent. To find the starting position, raise arms with relaxed bent elbows in front of the body at chest height. Soften the shoulders. Rest the right hand palm on top of the left hand. Both palms are facing down. Breathe in.

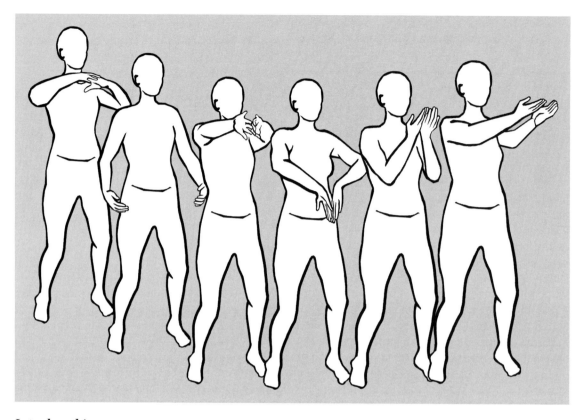

Lotus breathing.

2. As you exhale, release the arms downwards to the front and side of the body and allow them to softly release. Then in a swooping action bring them up to the side of the body in the front and towards one another. As the hands arrive at shoulder height at the end of the exhalation, touch the backs of the hands together in front of you.
3. At this point, begin to breathe in, drawing the hands down towards the navel keeping the backs of the hands together and deepening the knee bend. Rotate the downward pointing hands towards the heart and then outwards away from the body through the heart centre.
4. Hold for a moment before slowly releasing the exhalation, as you stretch the arms out in front of the body with palms cupped upwards. This action will bring the elbows closer towards each other. Try to extend the movement on the out breath for as long as you can.
5. Repeat several times remembering that in tai chi the emphasis is on the *flow*.

This exercise has the powerful effect of finding a physical form for the yin/yang breath exchange. The movement mirrors the growth of the lotus flower with its roots in the depths of the water, springing into bloom above the water. The lotus is a key symbol in tai chi as it contains both male and female/yin and yang qualities within.

Breathing into the Chakras
1. Stand in neutral with right hand resting in left palm and thumbs touching so that the hand makes a circle at approximately the dan tien area of the lower abdomen.

2. As you inhale, take the hands up to the crown chakra (*see* Chapter 4 for Chakra chart) keeping the palms and the thumbs together and slowly lower to the dan tien on the exhalation.

3. Try to visualize sending the breath to awaken this area. Repeat three times.

4. Repeat this action three times through each of the chakras in turn. Once you reach the root chakra your breath will have deepened considerably and you will feel both energized and calm.

Reflexology – Opening the Lung/Chest Area

In the previous chapter we looked at ways to work on the feet to open up the chest area. You can work in a similar way on your own hand to help stimulate the chest area to aid breathing. Just as the foot represents a map of the body, so too does the hand with the thumb correlating to the big toe and the fingers to the toes. The chest area is located in the top third of the hand that corresponds to the ball of the foot. At the bottom of this padded third of the hand lies the area corresponding to the diaphragm.

1. To prepare, rotate your wrists and stretch your hands.

2. Use the thumb caterpillar action to work across the lung area starting from the little finger towards the index finger. The fingers of the working hand should be supporting underneath the receiving hand.

3. You should do three rows working a little lower each time until you reach the diaphragm area.

4. Use the thumb walking action to work the throat area at the bottom half of the thumb on the palm side.

5. To finish, hook your thumb into the solar plexus that is located about a third of the way down the palm between the index and middle fingers. As you breathe in, press the thumb in and release as you exhale. Do this several times.

6. Now repeat on the other hand.

Shiatsu – Palming Down the Lung Meridian

The lung meridian is obviously connected to breathing so it is useful for performers to use this

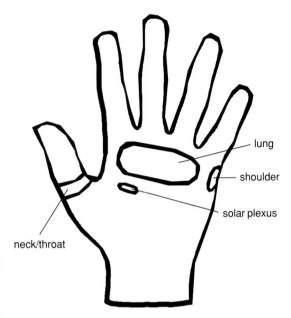

Reflex areas on the hand.

sequence to open up the chest and improve the quality of breathing and vocalization. The lung is also connected to the immune system and the skin, which is the first point of contact between the body and the world. Not only do we breathe through our skin but many imbalances are expressed through skin problems. In Traditional Chinese Medicine, the lung is the metal element and people who are strong metal types often have difficulty expressing emotions, which they hold onto. This can often result in shallow breathing.

The first lung point LG 1 is located between the first and second rib on the outer edge of the chest just under the collar bone, lying diagonally up from the armpit in a hollow just in from the shoulder. Feel this on your own body before locating it on someone else's. You should be able to place the heel of your hand in this area quite comfortably. The meridian runs down the inside of the arm on the outer edge (*see* Chapter 4).

1. Your partner is lying in supine with their arms at 5 and 7 o'clock positions, palms facing upwards.

2. Kneel at their head and centre yourself with your knees just above their shoulders. Place a scarf over their eyes to help them relax and forget about your proximity.

3. Take a moment to bring your energy into your hara and engage in sympathetic breathing.

4. Raise your hips to engage your hara and with a long back place each of your hands on your partner's LG1 points, one on either side of their upper chest.

5. Work with the breath to release on the inhalation and sink in gently on the exhalation. Your leaning pressure is directed slightly down toward their feet. Try to feel a sense of drawing up their energy to the surface. You are encouraging their breath to deepen so

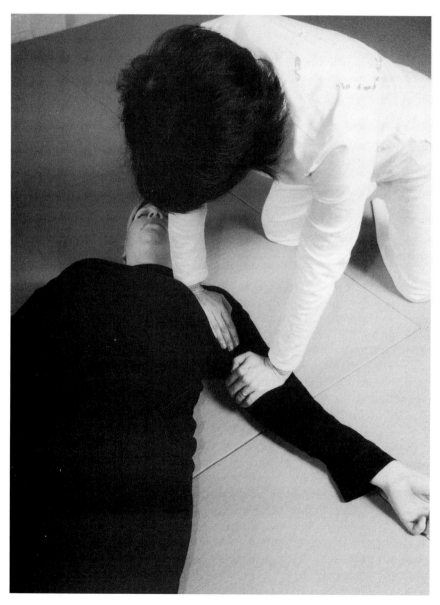

Palming down the lung meridian.

remain light on the inhalation and then as they exhale, sink in a little deeper – never pressing forcefully but gently releasing your body weight. Keep the cycle flowing from the hara. Remain there for 6–8 breaths.

6. Cross over your hands one at a time to maintain contact so that your right hand is now in the hollow below their left shoulder and vice versa. Lean in again to encourage deep breathing.
7. Release your left hand and move your body to their left maintaining your Mother hand on their left shoulder.
8. Palm down the outside edge of the upward facing arm towards the thumb using the Messenger hand to move and the Mother hand as stable in LG1.
9. Palm back up so that you can resume your position at the head with both arms crossed over LG1.
10. Now maintaining the left Mother hand below your partner's right shoulder, palm down the lung meridian on their right arm.
11. Resume position at the head and lean into LG1 on both sides for a few more breaths before slowly removing both hands on the out breath.

Working with a Roller
If you don't have the benefit of working with a partner, another useful way to open up the chest is to use a towel.

1. Roll up a small towel into a sausage shape, about the same length as your wrist to elbow. Now lie in supine on the floor and place the towel along the spine between the base of neck and the mid-spine (bra line). Lying on the towel will allow the upper back to open.
2. In time you will feel the vertebrae of the upper back beginning to unlock. If this feels too un-comfortable to start with, place a book under your head that you can then remove after a few minutes. Remember, as in Alexander work, twenty minutes will allow gravity to help the spine release (although ten minutes is still helpful).

Fish Vinyasa
The fish vinyasa works with a synchronized action of the chest and the breath mutually supporting one another. The previous exercise is a good gentle opener for this exercise.

1. Lie on the ground in savasana. Arms remain by the side of the body. Breathe in but do nothing.
2. Breathe out and as you do so raise chest away from floor and slide onto the crown of the head that remains in contact with the floor. Stay in this position as you breathe in.
3. Exhale as you slide your head away from you and lower the chest once more to the ground. Repeat sequence three times.

Having performed the fish vinyasa, you can rest and breathe in the full fish asana as follows:

1. Lie on the floor on a mat. Draw your arms together under your body and make fists of your hands that should be placed together under the sacrum. Draw your shoulder blades together. Relax.
2. Take a breath in and then on an out breath and keeping your fists and arms where they are, allow the chest to rise away from the ground, keeping the head in contact with the ground. Look behind you and breathe deeply. Allow the legs to stretch away from you. After several breaths, lower yourself to the ground and release the arms.

Partner Movement Work with Breath
The following movements have us listening to our inner impulses and closely connecting with our partner because we are virtually sharing breath throughout the physical exchange. The secret is in the releasing combination of movement with breath, and working with the support of a partner that allows a surprisingly sensitized exploration of self in relation to another. It is helpful to accom-pany these exercises with lyrical music.

There are three basic movements, the *incline*, the *tilt* and the *rotation* that are stimulated by the support of two hands on a partner's body. You need to be moving sympathetically and not imposing

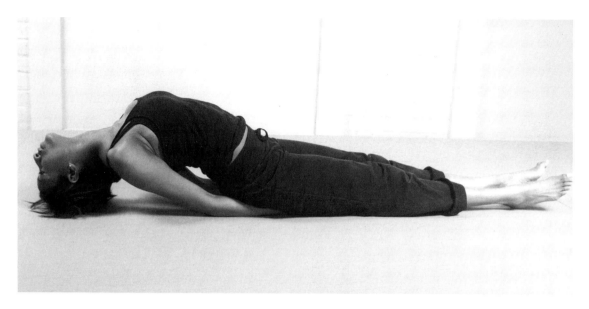

Fish asana.

the movement. Pairs should stand one slightly behind and to the side of the other.

Movement 1 – the Incline
1. Rest one hand lightly on the upper back/neck area of your partner standing slightly in front of you and place your other hand in front of their nearside shoulder (shiatsu point LG 1).
2. Breathe in and on the out breath, with the light contact of your hand on their back, your partner exhales, dropping the head and upper back forward and allowing the knees to bend slightly. Do not bend from the waist but keep your centres strong and stable, just softening the joints.
3. Inhale as you bring your partner back up to centre, straightening legs.
4. Exhale reversing the first action and allowing your partner to tip their head back and look up to the ceiling, using the support of your hands. The jaw may open.
5. Inhale as you return to centre. Repeat the two-way action up to a dozen times always remembering to exhale on the outward journey and inhale on the return to centre.

It is really helpful to work with another person, supporting your moves through each of these actions, but once you have felt the support of a partner in this exercise, it is possible to feel the movement on your own.

Movement 2 – the Tilt
This should follow on from the previous exercise.

1. Inhale and on the exhalation tilt the upper body to the right, bending knees and keeping in the same plane (not twisting forward or back).
2. Return to centre on inhalation and repeat to the left. Once the mover begins to respond they may well want to use their arms to help extend the quality of the action.
3. Person behind needs to judge where their hand contact will be most appropriate – it could be on shoulders, torso or upper arms of their partner, depending on how expansive the mover wants to be. Both partners soften and breathe, always connecting the breath with the movement. Repeat a dozen times.

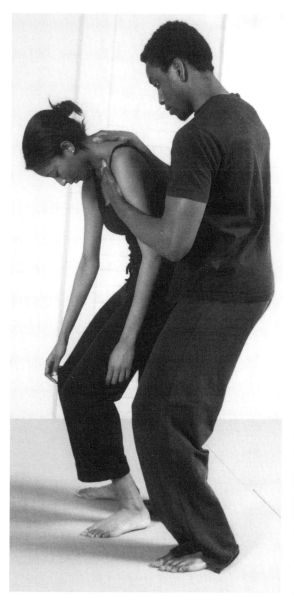

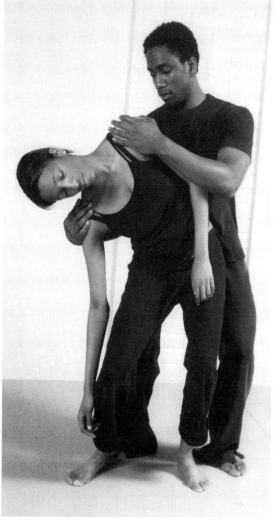

LEFT: *The incline.*

ABOVE: *The tilt.*

Movement 3 – The Rotation

1. Begin as before but the partner arm support may be on the upper arms of the mover. Inhale.
2. As you exhale, bend the knees, and rotate to the right.
3. Return to centre as knees straighten and you inhale. Exhale to the left, taking the movement to that side on bent knees. Repeat a dozen times.

With each of these three movements both partners should develop a rhythm and release into the movement as it becomes more comfortable and enjoyable. If partners are really connecting to one another, this becomes like a movement duet.

Improvisation – Combination of Incline, and Tilt and Rotation

Finally, allow the mover to move freely, improvising

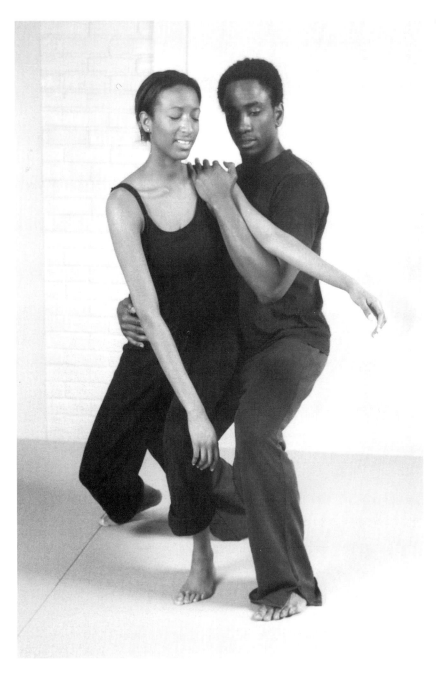

The rotation.

through all three of the above movements, following their own impulses and the direction chosen by the spine, to create their own breath-led movement score. Rather than initiating the exercise as before, the person behind now follows the mover and offers light contact only, sensing where the next movement is coming from on the edge of breath.

Out of Breath

Strong physical exertion can often make us breath-less. Although this is tiring it can also be exhil-arating. There are theatrical traditions associated with enduring extremes of physicality that bring a transcendent state. Probably the most famous was practised by the Polish director Grotowski, who would require his company to undergo radical yoga training and arduous breathing sequences as a prelude to rehearsal and performance. This work would leave the performers in a state of luminosity and with an improved readiness to seize on the creative challenge. Grotowski described this state as the 'via negativa'. The body is so exhausted and the normal defences so lowered that the performer becomes less guarded and therefore less likely to resist or respond with 'safe' reactions. In this purified state, responses may be more authentic and less edited as the predictable reactions burn off and a deeper level of experience is drawn on. Of course there are many ways of getting to this state. Some directors have used the practice of night running, whilst others use extended periods of energetic dancing to break down physical stiffness and mental reserve. You might try it for yourself by experimenting with the Ashtanga yoga sequence in Chapter 4, in which the breath fuels the powerful engine of the body or with Gabrielle Roth's Five Rhythms in Chapter 6.

Breathing and Voice

In general we tend to work with our voice within a very restricted range. While performers are often happy to work with movement in a very creative way, they can be surprisingly inhibited with ex-pressive voice work that goes beyond everyday speech. Even singing can be traumatic for those concerned with the quality of the sound and hitting the note correctly. The voice is revealing and may betray the emotional vulnerability of the vocalist if the breath is insecure. The production of the voice is totally dependent on breathing. But this works both ways; using the voice can help to improve the quality of breathing as it is stretched and extended in the creation of sound.

The body is made up of nearly 70 per cent fluid so that sound vibrations are very powerful. The

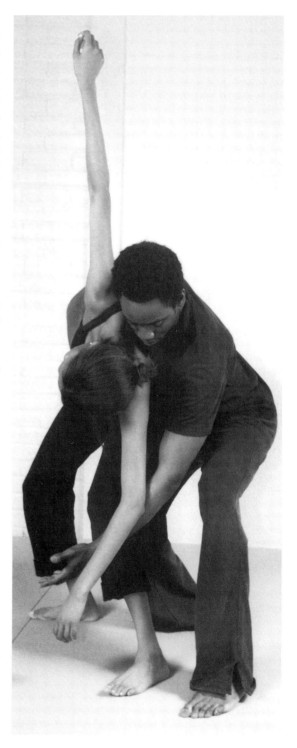

Breath-led movement.

ears connect with balance, rhythm and movement and are therefore linked closely to our nervous system. Sound waves can be used to harmonize with our organs or to create dissonances. We may be familiar with the singer who can break glass, and in medicine today sound waves are used to break down invasive matter in the body, such as kidney stones. Pregnant women listen to Mozart in order to soothe their babies in the womb, as loud, aggressive noises are known to be particularly damaging to young infants. Studies have shown how traumatized children survive by shutting down their hearing and consequently may have problems with being tone deaf. Harmonious tones can boost the immune system releasing endorphins, but most effective of all healing sounds is the resonance of one's own voice. The following exercises suggest ways of getting in touch with the resonators in the body and encourage playful ways of extending vocal range.

Sounding and Tapotement

Tapotement is a massage term referring to the loose wrist action of gently tapping the muscles to disperse tension, with relaxed fists, in a percussive action.

1. Your partner bends at the waist and hangs over with knees slightly bent, if hamstrings are stiff. Relax.
2. Make loose fists and gently tap your partner on the flesh around the shoulders, hips and thighs. Be careful to avoid direct contact with the spine but use the bank of muscles either side. Make sure you have relaxed wrists, hands and shoulders or your tension will pass through to the receiver. If necessary, kneel to reach lower extremities. Both breathe freely.
3. Your partner now allows the sound 'Ahh' to emit from the out breath in the process of being massaged. They should keep the sound strong and sustained, although they will need to draw breath between the sounds. The longer they keep the note going, the deeper the breath will be between sounds. Notice how the sound changes as the contact shifts around the body.

4. For the resonance to sound strongly the breathing needs to connect to the place where the tapotement is happening. You will hear this connection in the shoulders and upper back area, but encourage the breathing and sound to deepen by taking the massage further down the back, rather than just around the upper chest area.
5. When you have finished, place one arm on the back and the other supporting their belly as you slowly bring them to standing, uncurling their spine and bringing the head up last. Apply some firm strokes down the spine to help lengthen and ground. Your partner may feel a little dizzy so take time to secure them.

Belly-Laughing

So much of our voice production, in particular for females, is located in the upper chest and throat area, especially when the breathing is also restricted to this area. One effective way of getting a deeper resonance is to encourage sounds that emanate from a more guttural level. The belly-laugh is a very infectious way of rousing this sound. If you are in a group, it is useful to get someone to initiate the laughter that will spread until everyone is splitting their sides. You can try this by lying in a circle on the floor with your head in the lap of the person behind you and nominating one person to start the laughter off.

The Hum

A more gentle way of extending voice production is to lie on the floor and start a gentle hum. You will first of all feel the resonance in the nose and cheekbones. See if you can take it to various parts of the body by moving your hand to direct the sound. Sometimes the hum is quite difficult to feel in the lower body but if you alter the sound to an 'ahhhhh', you will be able to feel it further down the body into the far reaches of the abdomen. This is a good way of generating a strong ensemble feeling as you work to raise the volume and lower it to silence, responding instinctively to the group.

The Haka

Primal chants are a useful way of focusing and

Tapotement sounding.

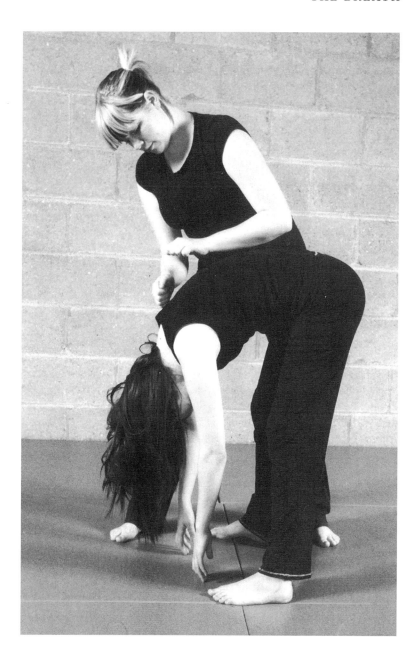

bringing up energy in group work. Many rugby fans will be familiar with the New Zealand tradition of the Haka, based on a Maori war chant. The sounds come from the centre of the torso, at the solar plexus, where Artaud located the anger zone of the body. It is the chakra that hosts our feelings of power and success. Explore the first few lines of this Haka. Breathe into the solar plexus before starting to sound and feel the strong alliterative effect of the hard consonants and the powerful 'a', sounded as in 'cat'.

Ka Mate! Ka Mate!
Ka Ora! Ka Ora!

It is often quite useful to use foreign languages to explore the emotional and expressive potential of speech that lies beyond sense. You can do this simply by using gobbledegook and see if you can still communicate your intention using tone, pitch, rhythm and emotional colouring.

Breathing and Chanting
One of the ways we can feel in touch with our breathing is through sounding the breath in a chant or mantra. People often shy away from chanting as they feel it is something mystical and suspect. The way to think about it is simply as an internal massage as the tiny vibrations created by sound warm up the inner muscles of the body. The interesting thing is that the voice then takes on a power that emanates from the body and is not necessarily controlled by the head. Chanting can release deeply felt emotions and vocal sounds stored in the body memory can take us by surprise. Our breathing improves as the quality of the sound resonates more powerfully and chanting can be a positive way of actually 'hearing' this improvement. At this point you would benefit from revisiting the chakra work in Chapter 4. This work encourages liberation of the performer's voice. Those who have never rated their ability to sing and think of themselves primarily as movers, often surprise themselves by the power and accuracy of their sounding capacity in this kind of work. Once you get used to the chakra sounds you can try sliding the chant from one part of the body/sound through to others and see how well your breath will support the transitions.

Notice how religions make use of chants in their calls to prayer that serve to open out the body to the experience of their faith. If you compare the religious praises contained in the Christian sounds of *Alleluia* and *Amen* with Muslim *azan* (call to prayer) *Allahu akbar* and the Buddhist divine abidings, *Aham avero homi*, you will notice how these all make use of very open vowel sounds similar to the sound 'ay' of the heart chakra.

Breathing and Meditation

Meditation is the practice of stillness of body, mind and spirit. It provides a haven from the 'busyness' of our cluttered minds that compulsively worry, plan and 'end-gain'. As we seem always to be activating our thinking without remission, leaping from one thought to another within a second, it is extremely difficult to turn off this mechanism. Yet you may remember moments in your life when you witnessed something extraordinary, like an amazing view, and were stopped in your tracks. The memory of this remains with you as you experienced a moment of stillness where all your senses, attention and body were united and you may have felt a sense of joy and serenity. You were present in the moment. This sense of inner calm and being at one with ourselves without the mind chasing ahead, is what we aim for in meditation. It is useful for the performer to be wholly in the moment, feeling grounded and cleansed which allows a return to rehearsal with enriched clarity and focus. The key to entering the meditative state is through the breath.

The Posture
In traditional yoga, the introductory asanas were always done with the express purpose of developing the body's strength and flexibility to the point where breathing and meditation could be practised with ease and with a sense of the body's lightness. When learning to meditate you may want to be in supine or sit upright in a chair with legs apart, arms free and palms resting. However, the optimum position is sitting with crossed legs in lotus position (with feet resting up onto the opposite thighs). This is very difficult to achieve for even seasoned practitioners, but the crucial aspect is to have a lengthened spine for maximum energy and breath flow, and any cross-legged position that you can hold comfortably will suffice.

An alternative position is to kneel with the knees apart and the feet together sitting on firm cushions or blocks; these supports create the right length in the spine. Whether sitting cross-legged or kneeling, there should always be a triangle of support at the base so that knees and feet are in solid contact with the floor and the torso is resting on the sitting bones with the hips above the knees. You may find that one knee is closer to the ground than the other. Again use a cushion or folded blanket to

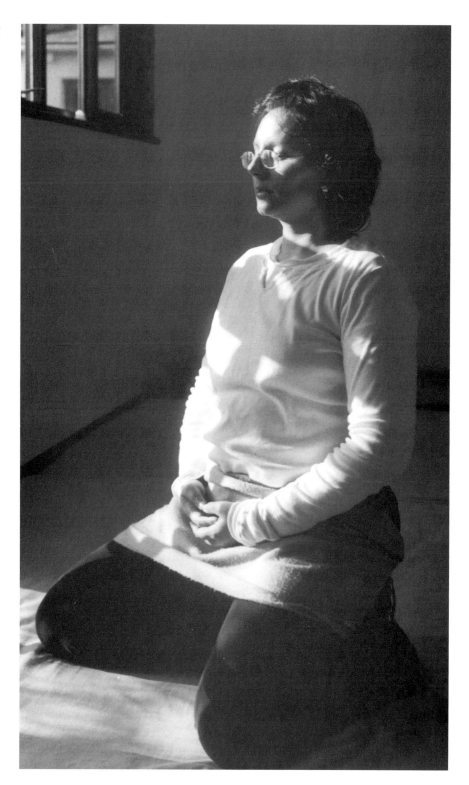

Supported kneeling for meditation.

support the raised knee so that it maintains contact with the ground. The hands lie palms up with the right resting in the left and the thumbs touching. They need to be placed at the dan tien area just below the navel, making physical contact with this source of energy. It is helpful to have a scarf wrapped around the hips to support the hands in this position.

The quality of breathing gained in this position is ultimately superior to that gained in a supine position – for one thing it is all too easy to drift off to sleep when lying down and breathing deeply. Just as we talked of the dynamic stillness of the performer, so meditation also requires alertness. With each in breath the spine lengthens and with each out breath the body softens and releases. It is important to maintain contact with the pelvis so that as the spine lengthens upwards it is also rooting itself downwards, from heaven to earth. A helpful visualization is to think of a plumb-line with the pelvis as the weight at the bottom. As you breathe, imagine the spine lengthening like a golden cord, the shoulder blades floating like rafts down and away from the neck. With each breath the shoulder blades feel freer and lighter, no longer tightly bound into the body.

Meditation and Breathing Visualizations
When first starting the practice of meditation it is important to give yourself time and space. You will not immediately be able to shut out your thoughts but you need to have a chance to separate yourself from the everyday world. The following meditation helps immeasurably to ground you and is a very good basis from which to begin. Use the same instructions until point 3 for all the following visualizations.

1. Make sure you are warm, quiet and comfortable in your sitting or kneeling position with your triangle base secure. Your hands should be resting at the dan tien. Close your eyes. Focus your breath on the belly area and observe the abdomen rising and falling with the breath.
2. Remember to think of your spine lengthening and rooting. Your body should feel light and

hollow as your mind centres in the abdomen on your breathing.
3. Now imagine a golden cube located in the middle of your abdomen. As you breathe in, it becomes more golden, as if alight. As you breathe out, the yellow cube holds its form but becomes like the embers of a fire, glowing. Stay with this visualization, allowing the image to transform if it wants to, but letting go of any extraneous thoughts. Keep the spine long, but feel anchored in the golden cube.
4. Try and stay in this position for 10 to 15 minutes, remaining mindful of your breathing. You may initially have difficulty imagining the cube and it may feel misshapen or lopsided. Just observe this, allowing your breath to keep visualizing the shape.

As you get more experienced and the spine becomes stronger, you will find it easier to stay for longer periods. You should try to practise this exercise daily.

The Smiling Belly
A very simple image is to think of a smile in the belly extending from hip to hip on the inhalation. This has the effect of softening the abdomen and deepening the breath. It also helps us to focus on the positive so that negative energy and thoughts that cause tension in the body, can be dissolved.

A Journey
Recollecting a place of security can, in the early stages of meditation practice, help encourage an association of peace and contentment with meditation. Imagine, therefore, that you are returning to a place where you have experienced joy. This may be a special location or a memory from childhood. Travel there and begin to imagine the smells, sounds and textures that surround you. Immerse yourself in the tranquillity of the space. Feel the edges of your skin tingling as you come into contact with the air.

Colours and Symbols
One of the most common ways to focus the mind in

meditation is to imagine a colour or symbol (yantra). The golden cube used earlier is the earth symbol that helps us ground ourselves. The colour green is often used as it is associated with calmness and nature. The deep colour of lapis lazuli blue is the colour most connected to healing in the Buddhist tradition so that immersing oneself in this state can bring about a strong sense of restoration, especially from fears. If you look back to the chakras you will see their association with colour, which may provide the basis for a meditation. Material symbols, such as elemental objects like candles and water, are useful in bringing the abstract thought in to the internal physical state. A very simple but effective one to generate a feeling of positive love toward someone is to take a flower and imagine it growing from the heart centre. Once you have done this, a simple visualization may be easier to achieve.

You may experience some strong emotions when meditating. Whilst it is important to recognize these feelings, try to keep a distance, using the discipline of your breathing to maintain a sense of detachment.

Mantra

The word mantra literally means 'tool of the mind'. A spoken phrase is repeated over and over having the effect of naming your intention and bringing it into the body. This is often used in Buddhist meditative practice but has become common amongst some psychoanalysts and healers who use affirmations to create positive thinking.

Dead Legs and Other Distractions

It is inevitable when you practise meditation that your nose will itch, your leg will go dead, your back will ache and you will be irritated by sounds that you never normally hear. This is part of the process and through this we learn to let go of the material world. Breathe through the irritation and keep reminding yourself that this will pass. Of course the other huge difficulty is not being able to instantly turn off your brain. The very time when you should be clearing it is when most thoughts seem to pop up. Treat it as though your head has a front door and as soon as the thoughts come in, don't try to close the front door but just sweep them out of the back door.

The End is in the Beginning

In some ways the practice of meditation is a precursor to all the preceding chapters, except that the one thing that appears to be the simplest and least challenging often turns out to be the most. Meditation can be seen as the culmination of bodywork, just as in yogic practice. The work enables you to be mindful in a way that enhances your awareness of everything around you. It awakens the senses, clears the mind and connects it to the body in a way that supports creative bodywork. It is therefore the very essence of holistic practice.

Having explored meditation you can now return to the beginning of the book and reexperience the exercises with a renewed simplicity of focus. After all, the best students are those who are prepared to begin again.

GLOSSARY

Alexander Technique: A system developed by Australian performer F.M. Alexander (1869–1955) to remedy body misalignment and improve body use

Asana: Yoga term for posture or position

Ashtanga: Dynamic system of yoga characterized by ordered sequences performed with corresponding breathing

Bandhas: A trio of energetic locks situated at the root, the lower abdomen and the throat, used particularly in Ashtanga yogic practice. Breathing techniques are used to unlock these bandhas thus releasing energy

Bilateral or contralateral: Movement pattern that involves a cross-patterning action of right leg with left arm and left leg with right arm – as in walking or baby crawling

Body armour: Name given to layers of muscle tension that encase the body

Body memory: Neurotransmiters within the muscle unlocking repository of subliminal memory

Body scan: Activity of passing the mind's eye over the body to detect subjective responses to body image

Body signature: Personal body language or movement vocabulary

Butoh: Post-war Japanese improvised movement form characterized by extreme slowness and distillation

Capeoira: Brazilian martial art form developed as a subversive dance by slaves in the seventeenth century characterized by acrobatic improvised movement anticipating opponent's intentions

Chakra: Energy wheel lying along the spine connecting the spiritual and physical worlds

Contact Improvisation: Improvised movement form developed in the 1970s primarily by Steve Paxton, characterized by highly sensitized partner interactions around a shared point of body contact, based on trust and counterbalance

Creative and Controlling cycles: Used in Five Element Theory to express the relationship between elements of Fire, Earth, Metal, Water and Wood

Cun or sun: Width of the thumb used as a measurement system for the whole body in Traditional Chinese Medicine

Dan tien: Energy centre located beneath the navel

Debauched kinaesthesia: Unreliable sensory feedback

Directions: Alexander's fundamental principles for movement: neck free, head forward and up, spine long

Emotional memory: Stanislavskian concept. Memory revived by activating sensations accompanying the original experience

End-gaining: Goal-oriented to the detriment of process

Experiential anatomy: Method shared by a number of practices, especially Bonnie Bainbridge Cohen's *Body/Mind Centering*, to familiarize ourselves with the body through strong visualizations

Feldenkrais: Therapeutic method developed by Moshe Feldenkrais (1904–84) based on rediscovering infantile movement to return the body to a state of ease and grace

Five elements or transformations: Chinese theory of understanding the cosmos and humans' relationship to it. Aspects of shiatsu and tai chi embody this theory

Five Rhythms: Therapeutic movement form developed by the charismatic American dance visionary, Gabrielle Roth

Habit: Ingrained tendency restricting spontaneous response

Hára: Area of the abdomen from bottom of the ribcage to the pubic bone seen as the power centre of the body in Eastern traditions. Important area for performers in learning to centre the body

Holistic: Therapeutic practice paying attention to the whole person rather than isolated aspect or area, characterized by a strong body/mind connection

Homolateral: Movement pattern involving one side of the body alternating with the other – as used by reptiles

Homologous: Movement pattern involving the top half of the body followed by the bottom half – as used by frogs swimming

Inhibition: Term with conflicting meanings. In the Alexander sense this refers to a moment of pause in which we prevent or inhibit our habitual response. In the Freudian sense inhibitions are blocks on our spontaneity

Iyengar: Celebrated yoga guru who developed an influential yoga system characterized by the execution of postures with a strict attention to detail

Ki or Chi or Qi: Term used in various eastern practices for energy in the body. Said to be generated through genes, environment and nutrition

Kinaesthetic: Sixth sense relating to intuitive awareness of ourselves as moving beings

Mantra: Sound used as a tool of the mind to assist meditation

Meridian: Invisible but palpable pathways of energy in the body, identified in Traditional Chinese Medicine and used in Shiatsu and acupuncture. There are twelve main meridians linked to body's organs and functions

Neutral body: Performance term used to describe a state of readiness for creativity from which personal mannerisms and tensions have been erased

Palming down: Technique used in shiatsu to describe two-handed continuous palm pressure applied with a stable mother hand and a moving messenger hand delivered by leaning perpendicular body weight over the body

Physical theatre: A recent development of theatre practice in which the body is paramount to communication

Pilates: Movement technique developed by Joseph Pilates (1880–1967) that focuses on developing core strength in the abdominal area

Prana: Term used in yogic practice referring to energy generated through breathing techniques known as pranayama

Primary Control: Alexander term for the critical head/neck relationship developed by his system inspired by observation of head-led animal movement

Prone: Anatomical position – lying on the stomach

Psycho physical: An understanding of how the body and mind affect one another

Savasana: Term used in yogic practice referring to the classic relaxation pose in prone position, often known as corpse pose

Semi-supine: Term used in Alexander Technique referring to the position lying on the back with knees bent and feet supporting legs, with support at the head

Shiatsu: Japanese system of touch therapy using the meridian system to balance and restore energy

Somatic: Literally meaning 'of the body' – generally used in relation to an awareness of the body

Supine: Anatomical position – lying on the back with legs extended

Tai Chi: Traditional Chinese movement practice characterised by soft joints and slow graceful, curving actions

Tapotement: Massage term referring to loose wristed, relaxed fist action applied in a percussive manner to fleshy parts of the body

Ujjai: Yogic breathing technique characterized by sibilant exhalation

Vinyasa: Yogic sequence of asanas threaded together on the breath

Yantra: Symbol used as a tool of the mind in meditation

BIBLIOGRAPHY

ALEXANDER TECHNIQUE

Alexander, F.M., *The Use of the Self* (Dutton, 1932).

Gelb, M., *Body Learning* (Aurum Press, 1991).

MacCallion, M., *The Voicebook* (Faber & Faber, 1988).

McDonald, G., *The Complete Alexander Technique* (Element Books, 1998).

Park, G., *The Art of Changing* (Ashgrove Press, 1989).

FELDENKRAIS

Alon, R., *Mindful Spontaneity* (Prism Press, 1990).

Feldenkrais, M., *Awareness Through Movement*, (Penguin Arkana (1972) 1990).

Feldenkrais, M., *The Master Moves* (Meta Publications, 1984).

TAI CHI

Al Huang, C., *Embrace Tiger Return to Mountain* (Celestial Arts, 1973).

SHIATSU

Beinfield, H. and Krongold, E., *Between Heaven and Earth: a Guide to Chinese Medicine* (Ballantine Wellspring, 1991).

Liechti, E., *The Complete Illustrated Guide to Shiatsu* (Element Books, 1998).

Masunaga, S., *Meridian Exercises* (Japan Publications Inc., 1987).

Masunaga, S., with Ohashi, W., *Zen Shiatsu* (Japan Publications Inc., 1977).

Ohashi, W., *The Ohashi Bodywork Book* (Kodansha, 1996).

YOGA

Iyengar, B.K.S., *Yoga* (Dorling Kindersley, 2001).

Mehta, S.M. and S., *Yoga: the Iyengar Way* (Dorling Kindersley, 1990).

Ozaniec, N., *The Elements of Chakras* (Element, 1996).

Scaravelli, V., *Awakening the Spine* (Harper Collins, 1991).

Scott, J., *Ashtanga Yoga* (Gaia Books, 2000).

CONTACT IMPROVISATION

Benjamen, A., *Making An Entrance* (Routledge, 2002).

Blom, L.A. and Chaplin, L.T., *The Moment of Movement* (Dance Books, 2000).

REFLEXOLOGY

Hall, N., *Reflexology – A Way to Better Health* (Gateway Books, 1991).

James, A., *Hands on Reflexology* (London, Hodder & Stoughton, 2003).

Norman, L., *The Reflexology Handbook* (Piatkus, 1989).

BREATH

Hanh, T.N., *The Miracle of Mindfulness* (Rider, 1991).

Manley, B., *My Breath in Art: Acting from Within* (Applause, 1998).

Turner, J.C., *Voice and Speech in the Theatre* (A. & C. Black, 1976).

BODY IN PERFORMANCE TEXTS

Artaud, A., *The Actor and His Double* (Calder and Boyars, 1970).

Boal, A., *Games for Actors and Non-Actors* (Routledge, 1995).

Callery, D., *Through the Body* (Nick Hern, 2001).

Dennis, A., *The Articulate Body* (Nick Hern, 2002).

Estes, C.P., *Women Who Run With the Wolves* (Rider, 1992).

Fralleigh, S.H., *Dancing into Darkness* (Dance Books, 1999).

Grotowski, J., *Towards a Poor Theatre* (Methuen, 1982).

Halprin, A., *Moving Toward Life* (University Press, 1995).

Hartley, L., *The Wisdom of the Body Moving* (North Atlantic Books, 1995).

Hodge, A. (ed.), *Twentieth Century Actor Training* (Routledge, 2000).

Marshall, L., *The Body Speaks* (London: Methuen, 2001).

Merlin, B., *Beyond Stanislavski: the Psycho-Physical Approach to Actor Training* (Nick Hern Books, 1993).

Newlove, J., *Laban for Actors and Dancers* (Nick Hern Books, 1993).

Olsen, A., *Body Stories: a Guide to Experiential Anatomy* (Station Hill, 1998).

Roth, G., *Sweat Your Prayers* (Newleaf, 1997).

Sabatine, J., *Movement Training for the Stage and Screen* (Backstage Books, 1995).

Stanislavski, C., 1984 *An Actor Prepares* (Methuen, (1936) 1984).

Todd, M., *The Thinking Body* (Dance Books, (1937), 1997).

Zarilli, P., *Acting (Re)Considered* (Routledge, 1998).

USEFUL CONTACTS FOR TEACHERS AND CLASSES

The Society of Teachers of Alexander
www.stat.org.uk
www.alexandertech.org
www.castat.ca

The Shiatsu Society
www.shiatsu.org
wwww.shiatsuprac.org

Feldenkrais Guild of North America
www.feldenkrais-method.org
Feldenkrais Guild UK
enquiries@feldenkrais.co.uk

Association of Reflexologists
www.aor.org.uk
www.reflexology-usa.org

Living Tao Foundation (tai chi)
www.livingtao.org.uk
www.livingtao.com

The Five Rhythms
www.5rhythmsuk.com
www.ravenrecording.com (USA)

Yoga
There are hundreds of centres offering yoga but
the following are from personal recommendation:

www.triyoga.co.uk
www.johnscottashtanga.co.uk
The Forge Yoga Centre
Totnes, Devon
01803 867444

Contact Improvisation
www.contactimprovisation.co.uk/london

INDEX

159